EVALUATION AND TREATMENT OF OBESITY

La Crosse Exercise and Health Series

Philip K. Wilson, EdD, Series Editor
Executive Director
La Crosse Exercise Program
University of Wisconsin-La Crosse

Epidemiology, Behavior Change, and Intervention in Chronic Disease, edited by Linda K. Hall, PhD; and G. Curt Meyer, MS

Evaluation and Management of Eating Disorders: Anorexia, Bulimia, and Obesity, edited by Kristine Clark, MS, RD; Richard Parr, EdD; and William Castelli, MD

Cardiac Rehabilitation: Exercise Testing and Prescription, Volume II, edited by Linda K. Hall, PhD; and G. Curt Meyer, MS

Cardiac Rehabilitation: Exercise Testing and Prescription*, edited by Linda K. Hall, PhD; G. Curt Meyer, MS; and Herman K. Hellerstein, MD

Evaluation and Treatment of Obesity*, edited by Jean Storlie, MS, RD; and Henry A. Jordan, MD

Behavioral Management of Obesity*, edited by Jean Storlie, MS, RD; and Henry A. Jordan, MD

Nutrition and Exercise in Obesity Management*, edited by Jean Storlie, MS, RD; and Henry A. Jordan, MD

The Elite Athlete*, edited by Nancy K. Butts, PhD; Thomas T. Gushiken, PhD; and Bertram Zarins, MD

*These five books were part of the Sports Medicine and Health Science series originally published by Spectrum Publications. Henry S. Miller, MD, served as the associate series editor.

EVALUATION AND TREATMENT OF OBESITY

Edited by

Jean Storlie, MS, RD
Research Associate
Institute for Aerobics Research
Dallas, Texas

Henry A. Jordan, MD
Director for Behavioral Education
King of Prussia, Pennsylvania

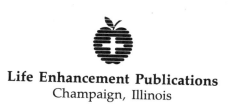

Life Enhancement Publications
Champaign, Illinois

RC
628
.E93
1987 Evaluation and Treatment of Obesity

Library of Congress Cataloging-in-Publication Data

Evaluation and treatment of obesity.

(La Crosse exercise and health series)
"Text is an outgrowth of the Obesity-Weight Control
Tract of the 1982 La Crosse Health and Sports Science
Symposium, sponsored annually by the La Crosse Exercise
Program, University of Wisconsin-La Crosse"—Foreword.
Reprint. Originally published: New York : SP Medical
& Scientific Books, c1984.   Originally published in
series: Sports medicine and health science.
Includes bibliographies and index.
1. Obesity. I. Storlie, Jean. II. Jordan, Henry A.
III. La Crosse Health and Sports Science Symposium (1982).
Obesity-Weight Control Tract. IV. La Crosse Exercise
Program (University of Wisconsin—La Crosse) V. Series.
[DNLM: 1. Obesity—therapy—congresses.   WD 210 E92 1982a]
RC628.E93   1987   616.3'98   87-22629
ISBN 0-87322-906-1

ISSN 0894-4261
ISBN 0-87322-906-1

Copyright © 1984 by Jean Storlie and Henry A. Jordan

All rights reserved. Except for use in a review, the reproduction or utilization
of this work in any form or by any electronic, mechanical, or other means, now
known or hereafter invented, including xerography, photocopying, and recording, and in any information storage and retrieval system, is forbidden without
the written permission of the publisher.

Printed in the United States of America

10 9 8 7 6 5 4 3 2 1

Life Enhancement Publications
A Division of Human Kinetics Publishers, Inc.
Box 5076, Champaign, IL 61820
1-800-DIAL-HKP
1-800-334-3665 (in Illinois)

1 66 47 46 2

Contributors

Andrew S. Jackson, Ph.D.   Professor, Department of Health and Physical Education, University of Houston, Houston, Texas

Henry A. Jordan, M.D.   Director, Institute for Behavioral Education, King of Prussia, Pennsylvania

Charles P. Lucas, M.D.   Obesity and Risk Factor Program, Harper-Grace Hospitals; Department of Internal Medicine, School of Medicine, Wayne State University, Detroit, Michigan

Michele Macedonio, M.S., R.D.   Director, Nutrition Services, Thomas B. Guilliam Associates, Twinsburg, Ohio

Cecelia Pemberton, M.S., R.D.   Chief Clinical Dietitian, Mayo Clinic, Rochester, Minnesota

Jean Storlie, M.S., R.D.   Research Associate, Institute for Aerobics Research, Dallas, Texas

Foreword

It is a pleasure to present the book, *Evaluation and Treatment of Obesity*, for reference and textbook use. The text is an outgrowth of the Obesity-Weight Control Track of the 1982 La Crosse Health and Sports Science Symposium, sponsored annually by the La Crosse Exercise Program, University of Wisconsin-La Crosse. With versatile faculty, topics, and attending professionals, the Obesity-Weight Control Track stimulated an effort to produce interdisciplinary resources on obesity.

Out of this effort, three books have been compiled and edited. This book, *Evaluation and Treatment of Obesity*, introduces an interdisciplinary, practical approach to obesity management. The other two books, *Nutrition and Exercise in Obesity Management* and *Behavioral Management of Obesity*, expand on the basic theories introduced in this book, providing in-depth information of value to the practicing professional. These three books apply the latest information from the fields of medicine, nutrition, exercise, and psychology to the problem of obesity. The information is intended to guide health professionals in the interdisciplinary management of obesity.

In 1983 the Obesity-Weight Control Track focused on controversial issues of theoretical and practical concern. The speakers from this track contributed their expertise to the compilation of two additional books. Thus, *Trends and Controversies in Obesity Research* and *Innovation in Obesity Program Development* will complete the series. Consider the five volumes a consolidated, comprehensive reference related to the growing, interdisciplinary field of weight control.

The co-editors and individual chapter authors of this book, and the entire series, should be complimented for providing the practicing health professional with a valuable book. Researching and writing this material has been enlightening and exciting to those involved; we trust its value to you will be similar.

Philip K. Wilson, Ed.D., Senior Series Editor
Henry S. Miller, M.D., Associate Series Editor

Introduction

Evaluation and Treatment of Obesity, is the first of a series of five books on obesity. The entire series is intended to (1) provide an understanding of the multiple factors that influence human obesity, and (2) apply this knowledge in developing comprehensive, rational approaches to weight management. A number of professional disciplines have made valuable contributions to the current understanding of human obesity. It is our belief that the complexities of this condition require the cooperation between and coordination of all these professions. Although the content of this series is divided into five books, it should be recognized that the material is interrelated and interdependent.

Consistent with this philosophy, *Evaluation and Treatment of Obesity* approaches obesity management from an interdisciplinary view. Representing the fields of medicine, nutrition, exercise physiology, and psychiatry, this book provides a general overview of the principles related to obesity treatment and evaluation. These concepts are expanded upon in *Nutrition and Exercise in Obesity Management* and *Behavioral Management of Obesity*. The last two books, *Trends and Controversies in Obesity Research* and *Innovation in Obesity Program Development*, are intended to address current issues of theoretical and practical concern. Within this comprehensive framework, the entire series approaches basic concepts in light of the problems that face practitioners at the "cutting edge" of obesity research and intervention.

Evaluation and Treatment of Obesity addresses two main issues: (1) why does obesity treatment present a problem to the health practitioner?

and (2) how do we begin to define and classify the nature of obesity in individuals? Chapter 1 discusses the scope of the problem in treating the obese. The complex mechanisms that influence energy balance and body weight are reviewed in Chapter 2, while the health risks associated with obesity are considered in Chapter 3. Chapters 4, 5, and 6 present methods for assessing obese individuals from three perspectives: health status, degree of obesity, and psychological influences.

The authors contribute not only their theoretical knowledge, but also knowledge based on considerable experience working with obese individuals. An attempt has been made to present theories, describe the practical applications, and discuss the "gaps" between theory and practice. This approach is intended to stimulate growth and innovation on the part of health professionals using this resource.

We hope that this book, and the entire series, will encourage health care professionals to face the problem of obesity intervention with practical and theoretical tools, as well as an interdisciplinary attitude. This effort can provide safe and rational alternatives to the myriad of untested, unscientific, at times unsafe, and ineffective programs that abound in our society.

Jean Storlie, M.S., R.D.
Henry A. Jordan, M.D.

Contents

Contributors   v

Foreword   vii

Introduction   ix

1. Obesity Treatment: State of the Art   1
    Henry A. Jordan

2. Regulation of Energy Balance   23
    Michele Macedonio

3. Medical Indications for Weight Reduction   43
    Charles P. Lucas

4. Clinical Assessment of the Obese Individual   71
    Cecelia Pemberton

5. Practical Methods of Measuring Body Composition   93
    Andrew S. Jackson

6. Psychological Factors Related to Eating and Activity Behaviors 113
    Jean Storlie

Index   153

EVALUATION
AND TREATMENT
OF OBESITY

Obesity Treatment

STATE OF THE ART

Henry A. Jordan

INTRODUCTION

The latest reports on the high incidence of obesity in the United States are alarming. Not only do they indicate that the average American is 18% overweight, but they also show that the incidence of obesity has continued to increase over the past decade. Coincidental to this increase has been a growing awareness that obesity is a major health-risk factor.

Albert Stunkard, M.D., stated in 1973 that obesity could be considered the greatest single preventable cause of death in the United States. There is growing evidence that obesity is associated with and may contribute to the severity of diabetes, coronary artery disease, and hypertension. Unfortunately, treatment advances have not kept pace with the increasing incidence of obesity. Not only are treatments often inadequate, but in the

Copyright © 1984 by Spectrum Publications, Inc., *Evaluation and Treatment of Obesity*, edited by J. Storlie and H. A. Jordan.

United States efforts to control obesity are often influenced by societal attitudes. There is a popular bias against obesity stemming from a cultural norm that manifests itself in the individual as a desire to be thin. In other words, concepts of beauty, handsomeness, chic, etc., are based on thin body-types, not obese body-types. As a result of this cultural conditioning, many people embark upon weight-control programs when indeed there may be no reason other than aesthetics to do so.

Thinness may be desirable, however, not only because it conforms to the aesthetic standard of a society, but because it may be related to good health. The relationship of obesity to disease is considerably more complex than first appearances. Therefore, we must use caution when considering who should be treated, for how long, and by whom. Although reports suggest and often strongly support a link between specific diseases and obesity, other studies indicate that not all obese individuals are at risk of either these specific disease states or increased mortality.

Because of the difficulties encountered both during weight loss and maintenance of lost weight, and the extremely high relapse rates, it may be very important to differentiate between benign and non-benign obesity. Dr. Lucas (Chapter 3) clearly outlines the medical indications for weight reduction. The social stigma attached to obesity, and the relationship between obesity and certain disease states clearly indicate the need for treatment. In fact, recommendations for weight loss have become almost automatic and universal, even for those individuals whose body weights are only slightly above the desirable weight tables.

Although there is evidence that moderate to severe obesity is associated with many diseases, there are no doubt overweight people—particularly the mildly obese—who have no risk for diabetes, hypertension or cardiovascular disease. Perhaps it is time that we evaluate obesity in relationship to both present and future disease, and begin to relieve some patients from the burdens of weight loss attempts. Our current preoccupation with thinness is creating a number of potentially harmful situations as more and more members of our society are using extremely drastic methods for weight control. Recent reports of the increasing incidence of eating disorders is probably directly related to the societal attitudes about body weight.

Even if weight loss is medically indicated for an individual it may be valuable to reassess our treatment goals. Commonly, the goals of treatment are to reduce weight to those levels set by the tables for ideal weight. Although the latest tables are more liberal than those of the past, it is unlikely that most obese individuals, especially those with long standing obesity, will be able to achieve such stringent goals. There is growing evidence that even modest weight loss may be beneficial in the control of diabetes and hypertension. A weight loss of ten to twenty pounds which can be achieved without drastic measures and maintained with only modest effort is more beneficial in the long run than a loss of forty to sixty pounds achieved through drastic measures only to be regained again.

Therefore, before considering any method for the treatment of a patient one must carefully assess both the necessity of treatment for that individual and, if treatment is deemed appropriate, what the reasonable weight loss goals should be.

In spite of the plethora of reducing techniques devised to manage obesity, to date treatment results have been poor and frustrating for both patient and therapist. Using diets, starvation, drugs, psychotherapy, self-help groups, exercise programs, and hormones, many patients are unable to lose weight, and of those who do lose weight, few sustain the loss for more than a year. Stunkard and McLaren-Hume reviewed medical management of obesity and reported in 1959 that all programs at that time were equally ineffective in their treatment of the problem [1]. Most studies showed that sustained weight loss is achieved in about 5 percent of cases. It has been over 20 years since this report and unfortunately, except in a few instances, those dismal results continue today.

Although a common outcome of most treatments has been the failure to produce sustained weight loss in all obese persons, each new method has had remarkable success with some individuals. At the present time, treatment is a hit-or-miss affair because there are no known indicators which predict the success or failure of a given individual with a given treatment. Hopefully, an understanding of the multiple causes and types of obesity will provide a key to determining success or failure of particular treatments.

In spite of these dismal results, there is little or no disagreement that effective treatment of obesity requires the achievement of negative energy balance through caloric restriction, increased caloric expenditure, or both. This means that the overweight individual must be skilled in calorie management, of both intake and expenditure. A recent editorial statement by the American Dietetic Association recommends that weight loss be achieved through dietary modification, alterations in eating behavior, and regular aerobic physical activity [2]. These recommendations constitute an excellent and time-honored prescription for weight reduction, but achieving these goals has been at best difficult for everyone and, in fact, impossible for most obese persons.

The reasons for such dismal statistics are perhaps best summarized by William Beaumont, when he said, in 1883, "In the present state of civilized society with the provocation of the culinary art, and the incentive of highly seasoned foods, brandy and wine, the temptation to excess in the indulgences of the table are rather too strong to be resisted by poor human nature" [3].

One wonders what Dr. Beaumont would say today, with modern day supermarkets, modern kitchens, and hundreds of new foods to choose from. After all, his statement was made three years before the creation of Coca-Cola, twelve years before the Hershey bar was invented, and twenty-one years before the hot dog was introduced.

Whether "poor human nature" is driven by biological or psychological forces, there is little question that many humans become obese easily and lose weight with great difficulty. As a result, the incidence of obesity in the United States has continued to rise, and for those individuals who have a disease related to their obesity, or have a risk of a future illness, successful treatment is important.

Although modern medicine has made such marked gains in the treatment of so many illnesses, the treatment of obesity remains imperfect. The continued rise of chronic diseases and the escalation of health care costs make effective and efficient treatment imperative.

In 1981 almost $287 billion was spent on health care in the United States, an average of $1225 per person. While the consumer price index climbed 8.9 percent, medical costs soared 15.1 percent. By far the largest proportion of costs were hospital costs. Hospital expenses in 1981 were four times the cost in 1971. The major illnesses, cardiovascular disease, stroke, diabetes, and hypertension may all be ameliorated and in many cases controlled by weight loss if the patient is obese. I repeat, though, that each potential patient must be individually assessed to determine if weight loss will have an effect on current or future illness.

THE REGULATION OF ENERGY BALANCE

Before reviewing the myriad treatments used in the management of obesity, it may be valuable to summarize those factors which enter into the regulation of energy balance. If we can understand the factors influencing the initiation of eating, the factors that influence the selection of particular foods, and the factors that are responsible for termination of eating, we can understand how a person's total food intake occurs. Eating behavior must be considered in the context of the world around us, our past experiences, and the biological processes involved.

Biological Determinants

There are numerous biological factors which trigger eating, influence the selection of foods, and influence the termination of eating. In and of itself, the set of biological processes involved in the control of food intake is immensely complex. These determinants, which have a primary genetic basis, tend to be stable over long periods of time. The biological factors determine the impact of other factors upon eating behavior. For example, a profound energy deficit produced by starvation may have a direct influence upon the type of food and volume of food ingested regardless of such factors as the food's palatability or cost, or the physical circumstances under which ingestion occurs. As was shown by Keys et al., during semi-starvation, prior food dislikes disappear, rates of ingestion are altered, and social amenities usually associated with eating change [4].

Some of the biological factors which must be considered are the role of taste, gastrointestinal factors, hormonal and nutrient levels in the blood, and the central nervous system.

If one considers man's evolution, the adaptability of eating behavior to changing environments is evident. There is much discussion in anthropology whether man is primarily a herbivore or carnivore. There are good reasons for this confusion as we have the long gastrointestinal tract of a herbivore yet the teeth of a carnivore. We retain a preference for sweets, a part of our herbivore heritage, and yet meat and fish are desired foods in a majority of world cultures.

Our origins go back at least 500,000 years. At that time, Homo erectus, a man who had a cranial capacity similar to our own, was a hunter and gatherer. He existed long before man had acquired the skill and knowledge to domesticate animals and raise crops. His ability to store energy was mainly in his biological capacity to deposit excess calories in his own adipose depots. He could also change his food selections from plants to animals. This enabled him to adapt to severe changes in environmental conditions, notably drought, famine, and extreme climatic alterations. We have preserved our omnivorous biological heritage, and we have also preserved our ability to adapt to changing environmental conditions. This biological adaptation to consume available food and efficiently put it into fat depots appears to be part of the biological heritage of Homo-sapiens and because of the bounty of food in twentieth century America this adaptation has run wild. The end result—millions of Americans with well stocked fat depots.

Much of the biological research has been directed at establishing differences between obese and normal weight animals and humans. Recent work on brown fat and ATPase offer hope for a future biochemical solution for obesity.

If we can begin to pin down differences in enzyme systems and metabolic pathways, then there may be hope for better diagnostic evaluation and treatments specific to various subgroups of obese individuals.

Macrosocial and Experiential Determinants

The second category of determinants comprise experiential, cultural, and familial factors. These factors also tend to be stable over long periods of time, but unlike the biological factors, most of these are determined primarily by the individual's early experiences with his environment. For example, early disturbances of psychological processes, as well as normal socialization processes, may determine early food preferences which then play a role in determining a person's life-long selection of foods.

Similarly, food selections are strongly influenced by broad cultural factors such as food taboos and the overall availability of particular foods in the society. The social and economic status of the individual and his family may also account for the type and amount of food generally available for consumption.

In every family, early learning experiences shape patterns of behavior which tend to be stable throughout a person's life. As each child has different genetic and environmental influences, so he develops different behaviors which enter into the regulation of energy balance and body weight.

In most instances, these learned behaviors result in the regulation of normal body weight. However, Ullman has outlined a number of ways by which a child may develop inappropriate eating habit patterns which lead to disorders in energy balance [5]. A common example of this process is when parental approval is given or withheld in association with the amount of food remaining on the child's plate. Through repetition of this process, the cue for meal termination is no longer an internal satiety signal but becomes the act of "cleaning the plate." In addition, food itself is a strong "positive reinforcer" as it satisfies physiological needs. Therefore, food may come to satisfy multiple emotional needs by being strongly and repeatedly associated with parental attention, comfort, and affection. Through this association, food may become a general way of coping with various emotional states. For instance, food can be used to reduce anxiety, alleviate pain, lift depression, relieve boredom, distract from loneliness, counter fatigue, or even enhance happiness.

Not only may parents actively teach inappropriate early eating behaviors and uses for food, but because the child patterns much of his behavior after that of his parents, the eating behaviors of the parent become incorporated into the repertoire of the child.

In addition to the early family experiences are the forces derived from the particular society in which we live. In the past fifty years, there has been a veritable explosion in the availability of food and food varieties for us to consume. Many of these changes stem from a variety of technological advances. Transportation has made available a greater variety of foods; today a typical supermarket may have 20,000 different items to choose from. Electricity has provided us with the means to rapidly cook and process food, and has provided light so we can eat at night. Canning and freezing allow us to maintain a greater supply and variety of food in our homes.

In the past 200 years, we have moved from a predominantly agrarian to an industrial society. Along with these changes came increased affluence, more money for food, and increases in leisure time. As our lifestyle changed, frequency of snacks increased, coffee breaks became routine. As we moved to office jobs and factories, eating away from home increased. In the past 20 years, there has been a rapid expansion of fast food restaurants, so that in the near future it is predicted that 50% of food dollars will be spent outside the home. Food advertising predominates in many magazines and TV shows. Children between the ages of 6 to 16 watch TV an average of 22 hours per week, and most children's advertising is directed at food and toys. The mass media now play a major role in the development of our food habits.

All of these changes in our society filter down to play an important part in defining each person's eating patterns. Because these factors are so prevalent, we are generally unaware of how different our present eating patterns are from those of the past. It should not be surprising, then, that an increased prevalence of obesity accompanies these macrosocial changes.

Determinants in the Immediate Environment

The results of these psychological, cultural, and familial determinants are further modulated by factors which are present in the immediate environment and the perception of the individual. Varying greatly from one individual to another, these factors lead to important differences in the behaviors occurring immediately before, during, and after ingestion. Each person, because of repeated experiences with these environmental factors, develops stable associations between the immediate factors and the behaviors involved in food intake.

Some of the more important aspects of our immediate environment which influence our food intake are time constraints, time of day, place of eating, immediate availability of food, food advertising, salient food cues, activities in association with eating, food palatability, and social aspects of the eating situation.

When the factors influencing food intake are viewed in this manner, it is clear that there is no single cause for excess adipose storage. Eating is one of the most complex behavior patterns encountered in medicine.

No simple formula for weight loss emerges from this analysis, since each aspect of individual eating habits and energy expenditure is deeply associated with lifestyle. What does emerge is the need, as the first step in treatment, to identify past and present determinants of behavior which contribute to high energy intake, low energy expenditure, or both.

INTERVENTIONS

There are various interventions and treatments that have been devised to attack each particular set of determinants. Modern medicine offers biological interventions for many illnesses and conditions, and a variety of these approaches have been directed at treating obesity.

Medications

For example, there are numerous drugs that have been developed to decrease appetite, based of course on the assumption that overeating is the result of unbounded levels of hunger. The initial anorectic drugs were the amphetamines and derivatives, but more recently several over-the-counter preparations containing phenylpropanolamine have been introduced. Phenylpropanolamine was judged by the FDA to be safe and effective for the treatment of obesity and therefore was released into the market as an over-the-counter drug. Phenylpropanolamine, a medication utilized in cold remedies for many years, is currently found in at least 64 over-the-counter preparations for colds and appetite suppression. It is difficult to test the efficacy of such a drug. The product is usually offered in combination with a package insert recommending a particular diet. The strong belief in appetite suppression by medication as a means of weight loss may produce a marked placebo effect. There is almost no evidence that anorectic medications produce long term weight control.

In addition to questionable efficacy of phenylpropanolamine, there is currently concern about the safety of the drug. In 1980 there were 10,000 contacts to poison control centers as a result of overdose of this particular drug. There are also reports of adverse reactions including psychotic reactions, and renal failure [6]. The FDA has asked the manufacturers of this drug to reevaluate what dose ranges can be deemed safe.

Perhaps the most important reason these drugs have limited value is the fact that many people, both lean and obese, ingest a considerable percentage of their calories in the absence of hunger.

Therefore the appetite suppressing agent is not affecting the very type of eating that may be most maladaptive.

Another class of drugs utilized for the treatment of obesity has been hormones. The most notable example is HCG, human chorionic gonadotrophin. This hormone must be injected and used in combination with a restrictive diet (often 500 calories a day). Frequent visits (almost daily) to the treatment facility are required. Controlled studies have shown no advantages of HCG injections over placebo injections, and the popularity of this treatment has diminished.

Another class of drugs are those that are meant to selectively block or interfere with the absorption of specific nutritional elements of the diet. The most common ones used in the past two years were the α-amylase inhibitors familiarly known as starch blockers. Recent research indicates that in humans the starch blocking agents do not block the absorption of starch calories any more effectively than placebo tablets [7]. Despite the lack of scientific evidence of efficacy in human beings, starch blockers are sold by the hundreds of thousands. This fact is further testimonial to the dieter's quest for thinness by any means, not evidence of drug potency.

In spite of the repeated failures of these biochemical interventions, the search for the magic pill continues. At least three U.S. pharmaceutical companies are attempting to develop drugs that would help people slim down by mimicking the effects of exercise. The pill would probably produce a low grade fever; possible side effects are currently unknown. These drugs are in early experimental stages; although they may hold the promise of effective weight control, their future potential is unknown.

Surgery

Another biological intervention is surgery. The initial surgical procedure utilized in the treatment of obesity was the ileojejunal bypass operation. By surgically rearranging portions of the gastrointestinal tract, large segments of the small intestine were bypassed and a malabsorption syndrome produced. Although weight loss was often dramatic, the long term adverse side effects of this surgery led to the development of the newer procedures directed at altering the anatomy of the stomach. Currently there are several variations of gastric surgery being utilized in the treatment of massively obese individuals. Although dramatic weight losses have been reported in many patients a recent editorial in the *Journal of the American Medical Association* indicated that failure rates for this surgery may be as high as 50% [8]. Almost all failures are due to one of three problems: the staples pull out, the new small stomach enlarges, or the entrance from the small pouch to the distal gastrointestinal tract stretches. Most often these problems are caused by the patient's eating beyond the capacity of the small pouch. These significant failure rates have been overlooked because few studies include sufficiently long-term follow-up. In view of these statistics this surgery should probably be viewed as experimental and be reserved for only the most drastic situations. Furthermore, operations should be performed only in institutions that are experienced in working with severely overweight individuals. Adequate long-term follow-up must be carried out to document both long-term efficacy and to discover the long-term complications. To subject patients to high risk surgery without adequate knowledge of long-term efficacy and complications would be unfortunate.

Jaw Wiring

A less drastic procedure is jaw-wiring. The teeth are wired together prohibiting usual eating behavior. This procedure usually produces weight loss, but most people gain the weight back rather rapidly when the wires are removed.

Purging

Although it is beyond the scope of this book to discuss anorexia nervosa and other eating disorders, there are two additional biological interventions that have been utilized to control body weight. Many individuals who have these disorders resort to the use of emetics and purgatives. These groups of agents produce vomiting or, in the case of laxatives, a rapid transit of food through the gastrointestinal tract. Many of the individuals who use these methods maintain body weight at normal or subnormal levels. The use of vomiting and laxatives for weight control should be strongly discouraged. These habits are socially disruptive and medically dangerous, and are very resistant to treatment.

Physical Activity

There is, however, one biological intervention that should be promoted. Physical activity is perhaps the most effective and important intervention necessary for successful weight control, and provides an increased expenditure of calories, suppression of appetite, and the potential for cardiovascular fitness.

SOCIOCULTURAL INTERVENTIONS

There are two major systems which have the potential for large scale intervention in the prevention and treatment of obesity, the media network and our educational system.

Media

The media, including magazines, radio, television, and newspapers has powerful effects on our eating and exercise habits. The power of advertising in shaping our behavior is staggering, but at the same time this network presents opportunities to deliver rational information to the consumer. Each professional must consider and take advantage of every opportunity to deliver legitimate information through every possible media channel.

Education

Our educational system also offers many opportunities to pass on information. We must begin to educate our children about proper eating habits, and particularly about proper physical activity habits. We must provide physical education programs that supply our children with activity skills for a lifetime. Competitive team sports provide great excitement and produce fitness in the participants, but when the season is over or school is finished the opportunities for continued participation diminish. Former athletes all too often become spectators, not participants. We must begin to promote and teach jogging, tennis, swimming, and walking as a means of providing activity for a lifetime.

Emphasis on activities for a lifetime are important not only for the overweight child and adolescent but for the slender child as well. Only one-third of the obese adults in the United States were obese as children. This means, of course, that two-thirds of them were thin as children. That fact alone underscores the need for programs aimed at lifelong habits during our school years.

Whether intervention is aimed at the media or in educational settings, the role of the professional must be twofold. The professional must (1) have expertise, and an ability to skillfully communicate that expertise; (2) the professional must provide a plausible and active role model. Learning occurs not only through active teaching but also by imitation.

DIETS

The final and probably the most universally used intervention is diet. Americans are in search of magical diets, and the use of even outlandish and at times unsafe diets is a testimony to the drastic measures that overweight people will go to in order to lose weight. The only books that out-sell diet books are bibles and dictionaries; generally at any given time the New York Times best seller list contains at least one diet book.

Almost all diet books offer promises on the jacket: "Herein lies an approach that is (a) completely new, (b) thoroughly tested, (c) based on old principles." Dieters will be taught to lose weight easily, without hunger or the "diet doldrums." At the onset the reader is given the scientific evidence for the diet's uniqueness or, if not available, a presentation of testimonials.

Most often certain foods or food groups are given magical properties in terms of fat mobilizing effects, metabolic differences, or magical combinations to promote malabsorption.

In most cases the scientific evidence has no basis in fact; testimonials are derived from the five percent of people who seem to be successful on any diet. Every diet has its remarkable successes, attesting to the fact that either each diet fits about five percent of the weight conscious population, or that at any given time five percent of the weight conscious population is ready to make substantial changes in their lives. Successful weight loss happens coincidentally with these other changes.

In spite of the high failure rates and unsound nutritional principles utilized in many fad diets, the public's desire for quick, easy loss continues, and the market for diet books continues strong in spite of these abysmal statistics. However, like late-model automobiles most have limited sales lives. They appeal to the consumer who is looking for the latest model, and the most successful are fads. The "Beverly Hills Diet" was recently the latest rage, "Pritikin" and "Scarsdale" swept the country a few years earlier, "Atkins" and "Stillman" preceded these, and "Taller" came before that. As the fad fades, the weight returns, to be taken off again with the next diet.*

A nutritionally balanced, calorically restricted diet may be important for the treatment of obesity, but the success rate of even medically sound dieting is low. If used, a diet must be offered in the framework of a comprehensive program. Each element of the program is addressed in the remainder of this book. The major consideration, I believe, is to provide our patients with a lifetime of options, not limitations.

Probably the most common mistake made in dietary management, regardless of treatment regimen, is to try to treat all obese persons alike. While our knowledge of the controls of eating behavior and dietary selection, and physical activity is far from complete, it is apparent at this time that a variety of factors can lead to improper eating habits, food selection, and depressed levels of physical activity. Treatment must reflect individual differences with respect to these factors as well as the person's attitudes, interpersonal relationships, and the quality of their lives.

*Fad diets are discussed more fully in P. Hodgson, Review of popular diets. In *Nutrition and Exercise in Obesity Management*, edited by J. Storlie and H. A. Jordan (New York, Spectrum Publications, 1984).

BEHAVIORAL COGNITIVE APPROACHES

Dieting, per se, is avoiding the issue. A person on a diet avoids the very foods that have caused difficulty in the past, and therefore does not learn to deal constructively with these foods. What is indicated is a treatment program aimed at helping people to learn to eat differently, to move differently, and to develop a way of eating that they can live with for the rest of their lives.

In order to promote adaptive eating and activity patterns, however, it is not enough to offer only simple behavioral prescriptions. It is also necessary to explore the psychological and attitudinal determinants of these behaviors and the psychological consequences of behavior change. Thus one must consider the general psychological issues which are often intimately intertwined with the eating behavior and lifestyle of the obese. These are psychological factors which (1) effect the development of obesity, (2) result from being obese, (3) result from losing weight or attempting not to be obese and, finally, (4) occur after an individual has successfully lost weight. (See Storlie, Chapter 6, for further discussion.) It should however, be made clear that not all obese individuals experience psychological problems.

Bruch has described numerous cases of intrapsychic and often intrafamilial psychopathology that accounted for a patient's obesity [9]. Even so, nobody has found a uniform family constellation specific for obesity. Therefore, it would be a mistake to assume that psychopathology is involved in all cases of obesity. Although Richardson hypothesized in 1946 that obesity was a manifestation of neurosis, most studies since then have found this concept elusive [10]. Most attempts at defining an obese personality type or personality traits common to all obese individuals have failed. Although it can be stated that psychopathological factors may cause the development of obesity in some people, not all obese persons are obese as a result of psychological problems. More important than traditional psychopathology are psychological concomitants of learning which result from our everyday experiences, and which come to influence our eating and activity patterns.

The second major category of psychological factors are those which result from being obese. In this area one must be careful to differentiate problems arising from intrapsychic conflicts from those problems arising from conflict between the obese individual and a society which places a high value on thinness.

The majority of psychological difficulties seen in obese individuals fall into this category. Problems arising from society's negative view of obesity are a result of and not the cause of the obesity. Widespread recognition of these problems has probably given rise to the common assumption that obesity has its roots in emotional instability. Obese individuals, however, cannot be viewed in isolation from the themes that underlie many aspects of their daily lives.

There is ample evidence that American society is significantly prejudiced against the obese individual. Our preoccupation with thinness has led to intense pressures on the obese to conform to this arbitrary "norm." As Cahnman has pointed out, obese individuals in our society are at a triple disadvantage: First, they are discriminated against; second, they are made to feel they deserve such discrimination; and third, they come to accept their treatment as just [11]. The stigma attached to obesity leads to low self-esteem, a variety of negative distorted attitudes about food, doubts about capabilities, impairment of interpersonal relationships, and social isolation.

The American ethic dictates that we be productive, competent, rational, and most importantly, in control of ourselves and our lives. We live in a world that emphasizes achievement and constant striving for success. However, we most often gauge our success not by our own estimates of competence in work, but by our perception of the evaluations made by others. Obesity in this context is viewed as evidence of a lack of control and a lack of success. Ultimately, the public views the obese individual as one who has not worked hard enough and is lacking in "character."

Allon, in an excellent review of the stigma attached to obesity [12], organizes the discrimination against obese individuals into four broad areas. First, from a religious perspective, obesity is regarded as the result of gluttony, one of the "seven deadly sins." This concept is mirrored in the attitudes prevalent among the obese themselves as they attempt to struggle with their problems. One frequently hears confessions of sin, testimonials to virtuous self-denial, and expressions that sins must be expiated through suffering and repentance. The eating of "forbidden" foods is followed by guilt, shame, and remorse.

A second perspective outlined by Allon is the medical view that obesity is a disease. In this model, the obese individual is regarded as sick—physiologically, psychologically, or both. Although there is little disagreement that obesity is associated with diabetes, hypertension, cardiovascular abnormalities, and a variety of other medical conditions, labeling the obese individual as sick is of no therapeutic value, and is often counterproductive.

In a third perspective, obesity is viewed as a crime. Here, overeating is viewed as a felony or misdemeanor, and the obese individual is met with public scorn for his or her wrongdoing. Overeating is perceived as breaking an unwritten "law" against excessive behavior, as reflected by the term "cheating" on a diet.

These first three perspectives are outlined in Figure 1. The fourth and final view of obesity is in the context of cultural aesthetics. Here, obesity is viewed as a form of ugliness. The fashion industry underscores this negative concept by highlighting fashionable apparel for thin persons, but provides limited choices of color or style for the obese. Even the ads for styles for the "large" woman picture thin, well-proportioned females.

When one considers the labels "sick," "ugly," "sinful," "criminal" as applied to the obese individual, one can understand why obese individuals may develop severe emotional problems.

The labeling of obesity as a disease, sin, or crime leads quite naturally to a labeling of methods of control. The traditional diet then becomes either a cure for the disease, a part of repentance and atonement for the sin, or a punishment to fit the crime. Little wonder that obese individuals are so ambivalent in their feelings toward dieting.

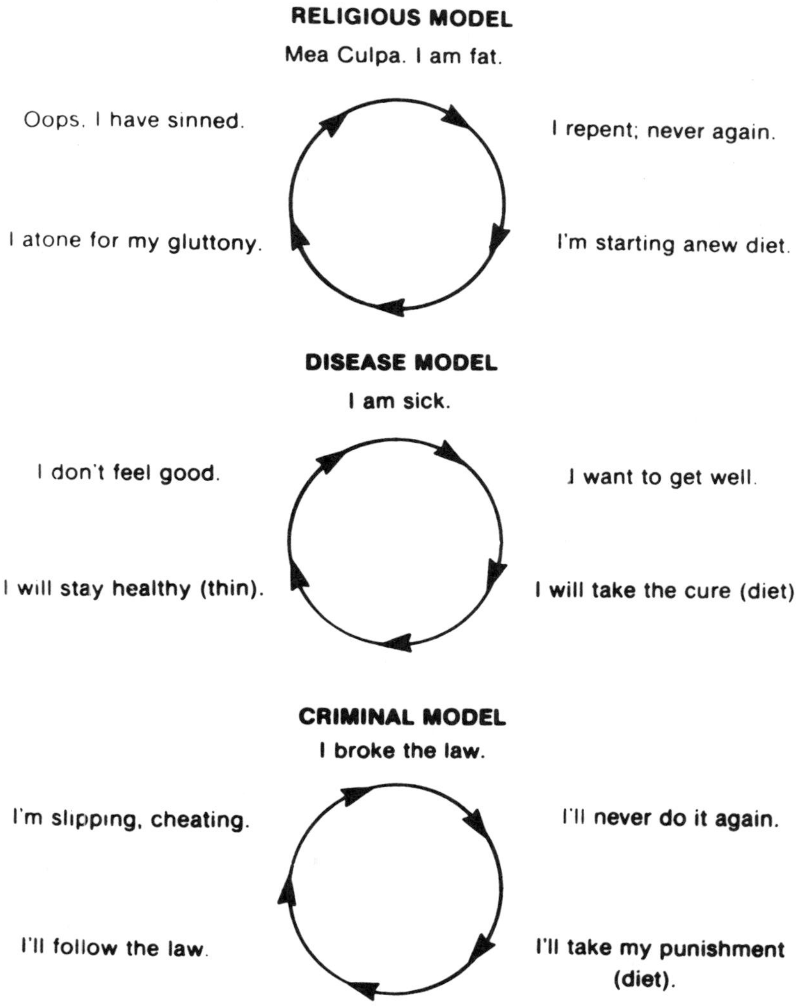

RELIGIOUS MODEL

Mea Culpa. I am fat.

Oops. I have sinned.

I repent; never again.

I atone for my gluttony.

I'm starting anew diet.

DISEASE MODEL

I am sick.

I don't feel good.

I want to get well.

I will stay healthy (thin).

I will take the cure (diet)

CRIMINAL MODEL

I broke the law.

I'm slipping, cheating.

I'll never do it again.

I'll follow the law.

I'll take my punishment (diet).

Figure 1. In our society, obesity is often regarded as a sin, disease or crime. For example, in the religious model, the cycle starts with "mea culpa," "I am guilty" and goes on to "I have sinned. I have eaten 'bad foods." "I have gained weight." The next stage is repentance followed by dieting and atonement. Inevitably, the dieter yields to temptation and sins again. Reprinted with permission of the author from *The Doctor's Calories-Plus Diet*.

Table 1. Some Foods and the Moral Values
Attached to Them

Sinful Unhealthy Illegal Foods	Holy Healthy Legal Foods
sugar	saccharin
carbohydrates	protein
ice cream	yogurt
bread	salad
candy	celery
pizza	tuna
mayonnaise	cottage cheese
bacon	turkey
butter	margarine

As a result of the labeling of obesity as a disease,
sin or crime, foods are often dichotomized. The
"bad" foods on the left are delightful to eat, but
may produce negative after-reaction. The "good"
foods on the right produce positive after-reaction.

The stigma attached to obesity is also transferred to the
foods people eat. Foods are regarded not only as nutritional
supplies for the body but the society gives them moral values
as well, as indicated in Table 1. Foods are viewed as good or
bad, healthy or unhealthy; thus, a person's self-esteem may be
raised or lowered by the ingestion of "good" or "bad" foods,
respectively. Treatment then must be directed as much to an
understanding and amelioration of the psychological difficulties
of the obese patient as to weight loss.

Unfortunately, there are no simple solutions, neither behavioral or medical, because there are no simple lives. Our eating
behavior, our physical activity, the maintenance of our energy
balance, is intimately wrapped up with the way we live our lives.
Americans in general live lives that are conducive to overeating
and inactivity. I think that the behavioral cognitive approach
stressing both behavior and attitude change currently offers
our greatest hope. The development of better psychological
and physiological assessments is imperative for improving
existing therapies. Through increased understanding of the multiple determinants of obesity we should be able to select the

appropriate treatment or treatment combinations suited for each individual.

Regardless of what methods are used, they must be imbedded in a program that takes into account people's lifestyles, their personalities, and the quality of their lives.

REFERENCES

1. Stunkard, A. J., and McLaren-Hume, M. The results of treatment for obsesity. A review of the literature and report of a series. *Arch. Intern. Med. 103*:79, 1959

2. Anonymous. Editorial: Nutrition and physical fitness. A statement by the American Dietetic Association. *J. Am. Dietetic Assoc. 76*:437, 1980.

3. Beaumont, W. *Experiments and Observations on the Gastric Juice and Physiology of Digestion.* New York, Dover, 1959.

4. Keys, A., Brozek, J. Henschel, A., Mickelson, O., and Taylor, H. L., *The Biology of Human Starvation* (2 vols). Minneapolis, University of Minnesota Press, 1950.

5. Ullmann, L. P., Krasner, L. *Behavior Influence and Personality.* New York, Rinehart and Winston, Inc. 1973.

6. Dietz, A. J. Amphetamine-like reactions to phenylpropanolamine. *JAMA, 245*:601, 1981.

7. White, P. L., and Selvery, N. Nutrition and the new health awareness. *JAMA, 247*:2914, 1982.

8. Reed, M. Editorial. Bad and good news on gastroplasty. *JAMA, 248*:277, 1982.

9. Bruch, H. *Eating Disorders: Obesity, Anorexia Nervosa and the Person Within.* New York, Basic Books, 1973.

10. Richardson, H. B. Obesity as a manifestation of neurosis. *Med. Clinics N. Am. 30*:1187, 1946.

11. Cahnman, W. J. The stigma of obesity. *Sociology Quar. 9*:283, 1968.

12. Allon, N. The stigma of overweight in everyday life. In: *Obesity in Perspective.* Washington, D. C., Government Printing Office, 1973.

2

Regulation of Energy Balance

Michele Macedonio

INTRODUCTION

Preliminary to any discussion of weight control is a definition of terms. Although often used synonymously, overweight and obesity are not identical. Overweight denotes an excess of body weight relative to standards for height, whereas obesity refers to a surplus in body fat. Body fat is the quantity of triglyceride and other fats which the body contains and is the major constituent of adipose tissue.

"Obesity tissue" is a term, introduced by Keys and Brozek [1], chemically describing the mass composed of fat, protein and other cell solids, and water, resulting from excessive caloric intake.

Most discussions of weight control begin with investigations into the phenomenon of obesity. A review of the research on the factors influencing obesity [2] reveals a diverse focus

Copyright © 1984 by Spectrum Publications, Inc., *Evaluation and Treatment of Obesity*, edited by J. Storlie and H. A. Jordan.

ranging from social and psychological influences to metabolic functioning. The ultimate purpose of this review is to provide the clinician with a rationale for designing weight management plans. Research into physiologic, dietary, and social/environmental determinants of body weight is interpreted and applied to the development of strategies for effective weight control.*

PHYSIOLOGIC FACTORS AFFECTING WEIGHT

If one ascribes to the law of conservation of energy for animal metabolism, body weight is the end result of energy consumed versus energy expended. More specifically stated by Brody, "The energy equivalent of work performed by an animal, plus the maintenance energy of the animal, plus the heat increment of feeding must equal the energy generated from the oxidation of nutrients" [3]. Physiologic investigations into obesity have attempted to unravel the mechanisms of the transfer of energy within the body. Research in this area has been prolific, revealing data which challenge past speculations, clarify some old theories, and provide the basis for new theories.

Genetics

Is one predisposed to obesity or leanness? It does not take detailed scientific investigation to discover that there are familial trends in weight. The question is over the sources of the these trends. What evidence exists to support the theories of genetic endowment as a significant factor in the development of obesity? And what part does the family environment play? Although limited, research into the genetic factors affecting weight supports a possible genetic link [4]. Studies on twins indicate that heredity contributes to weight into adulthood when environmental factors all but disappear. Adoption studies, although constrained by confounding factors, further suggest that heredity may play a role in the development of obesity [5].

*See also M. Macedonio, Nutritional management of the obese individual. In *Nutrition and Exercise in Obesity Management*, edited by J. Storlie and H. A. Jordan (New York, Spectrum Publications, 1984).

Statistics from the Ten State Nutrition Survey [6] support the concept of environmental influence on weight. Garn and Clark [7], in reviewing this data, conclude that the environmental influences of the family are largely responsible for familial resemblance. Given a genetic propensity toward obesity, environmental conditions, e.g., food intake and activity patterns, may override such a predisposition. As illustrated by Mayer [8], genetically obese mice can be kept thin by controlling kilocalories and increasing caloric expenditure. The familial effect on weight, then, is two-fold: both genetic and environmental.

Mechanisms of Weight Regulation

Medial Hypothalmus. Weight is under homeostatic control involving both internal and external energy-related stimuli. The brain is the central regulatory center which integrates neural and hormonal signals. Research has attempted to trace the regulatory processes of the brain which direct the physiology and psychology of weight regulation. Laboratory experimentation mainly with rats is focused on the hypothalmus, the control center for lipostatic, thermostatic, and glucostatic mechanisms thought to control energy homeostasis and the motivation to eat. Brain research on obesity has been conducted using four major approaches: (1) brain lesions, (2) neuropharmacological manipulation, (3) brain stimulation, and (4) neural recording.

Lesions of the ventromedial hypothalmus have been shown to induce hyperphagia which leads to obesity. Interestingly, not all VMH-lesioned animals will overeat. Teitelbaum [9] demonstrated that rats made obese prior to lesioning will not overeat after being lesioned. If force-fed to become super obese, rats will undereat until they reach their prior level of obesity [10]. The effect of this syndrome is not simply one of overeating, but eating to maintain a higher level of fat, thus, body weight.

Hyperfunction of the vagus nerve is another observed effect of VMH-lesions, suggesting a causal effect of increased gastric function on hyperphagia. Studies indicate that the medial hypothalmus involves both internal and external signals. The lesions affect hormonal secretions, particularly pituitary hormones, growth hormone, insulin, and inhibit gastrointestinal functions.

When food intake is matched for control and lesioned rats, the lesioned rats lay down some excess fat [11], indicating that hyperinsulinemia or some other metabolic effect causes a higher body weight on a normal food intake. Holding insulin levels constant (either surgically [12] or pharmacologically [13]) in medial hypothalmic lesioned rats produces mild and marked hyperphagia, respectively. The conclusions to be drawn are that medial hypothalmic lesions directly cause hyperinsulinemia and hyperphagia, and although the results occur independently of one another, they indirectly facilitate each other. Put plainly, this syndrome results in a vicious cycle of fat storage.

The entire picture involving the medial hypothalmus is not fully understood. Lesions of the medial hypothalmus affect humoral functions as well as insulin production. By altering pituitary hormone-releasing factors, lipolytic and lipogenetic hormone release may increase lipogenesis and obesity. Based on research to date, it can be concluded that damage to the medial hypothalmus results in "cellular overfeeding" from hyperinsulinemia and "behavioral overfeeding" due to hyperphagia [14].

Lateral Hypothalmus. A lateral lesion syndrome, in many respects, is the converse of the medial lesion syndrome [14]. The lateral lesioned rat subnormally responds to sensory cues, i.e., touch, taste, and odor, in contrast to the heightened sensory sensitivity in the medial hypothalmic lesioned rat. A low weight is maintained in lateral hypothalmic lesioned rats; obesity is maintained in medial hypothalmic lesioned rats.

The alteration in the sensory response of lateral hypothalmic lesioned rats is relative to the sensory control mechanism in the lateral hypothalmus. In addition to reducing sensory response to food, lateral lesions augment satiety. If the medial hypothalmus is intact, laterally lesioned rats actively reject food. With both lateral and medial damage, rats are more likely to accept food [15].

The functions of the lateral hypothalmus are the opposite of the functions of the medial hypothalmus and, thus, the two are mutually inhibitory. Whereas damage to the lateral hypothalmus may cause reduced food intake due to a subnormal response to both internal and external cues, if coupled with some medial damage, a rat may still maintain a normal body weight.

Fat Cells

Adipose tissue is a depository of stored energy. It is composed mainly of fat (approximately 90% or more), some protein, and water. The predominant fat in adipose tissue is triglyceride which is made up of free fatty acids and glycerol. Cholesterol and phospholipid account for approximately 0.16% and 0.15%, respectively. Since the main function of adipose tissue is to store and release fat, adipose tissue mass has wide variations in size—within the same individual and between individuals. Not only does the size of adipose tissue mass vary, but so, too, do the number and size of individual fat cells.

Some of the popular theories about the regulation of body weight suggest that total energy reserves are regulated [2,12]. Kennedy [16] hypothesized that food intake is under "lipostatic" control; that is, the hypothalmic satiety mechanism responds to the amount of fat in the depots. Subsequent research lent support to this theory [17,18]. However, later studies shed new light on the subject by indicating that the regulatory mechanism is the weight of individual fat cells rather than the total body fat [19,20]. Further animal study supports the hypothesis that once the "maximum cell size is reached in different depots, proliferation of fat cells may take place for further fat storage." This information challenges the "critical period" concept that cell proliferation occurs in infancy and ceases sometime in early life. From then on, an increase in cell mass was thought to be a result of individual fat cell hypertrophy. The basis for this theory comes largely from the investigations of Hirsch and Knittle [21], who report a three-fold increase in fat cells during the first year of life and a continual gradual increase throughout childhood. Hager and Sjostrom et al. [22], found the opposite. During the first 12 months of life, the increase in adipose tissue mass was due mainly to an increase in the size of individual fat cells with no change in fat cell number. The discrepancy of results between the two groups of investigators may be due to the method of quantitating fat cells. Using an automated method of counting fat cells, Hirsch and Knittle may have overestimated fat cell size in infants, leading to the conclusion of rapid cell proliferation during the first 12 months [23].

Both animal [19,24,25] and human [22] investigations support the theory of "maximum cell size" in the regulation of fat cell number. This theory holds that once the "maximum cell size" is reached, proliferation of fat cells may take place for further fat storage. Thus, fat cell number can increase at any age with the attainment of a fat cell size which triggers cellular hyperplasia, but it cannot be reduced by weight loss.

Bjorntrop and Sjostrom [26] found a positive correlation in the lower ranges of body fat between fat cell weight and total body fat. In higher ranges of body fat, the correlation was between the number of cells and total body fat. These results led the Swedish investigators to postulate two types of obesity: a hypertrophic obesity characterized by increased fat cell size, and hyperplastic obesity which results from increased fat cell number. The work of Hirsch and colleagues [27] support this theory. Thus, all obese individuals have hypertrophic obesity, and those with hyperplastic obesity (above 30 kg/66 lb) have hypertrophic obesity as well [26]. Hypercellularity, although associated with early onset of obesity [21,27,28], occurs in some individuals with late onset obesity and is not present in some patients who become obese early in life [27,28]. The metabolic associations with fat cell weight show a positive correlation between fat cell weight and plasma insulin levels [26] and hypertriglyceridemia [29,30]. Glucose oxidation, synthesis, and triglyceride, as well as lipolysis and release of fatty acids are elevated in large fat cells compared to smaller ones. Due to a hyperlipolytic hyperinsulinemic condition with enlarged fat cells, a tendency toward increased plasma triglycerides occurs.

In response to treatment [31], positive correlations exist between the number of fat cells in relation to weight loss, rate of weight loss, and rate of regain. Negatively correlated are the number of fat cells and the duration of maintained weight loss. Clearly, hypercellular obesity is more difficult to treat than the hypertrophic form. Since in some individuals fat cell number increases when weight is elevated over previous levels, yet fat cell number has not been shown to decrease with weight reduction, the goal of treatment in severe cases may be more realistically set if aimed at the prevention of further gain. This also has direct application toward preventive measures of weight control.

Set Point Concept of Weight Regulation

The term "set point" is becoming the weight control catchword of the 1980s, supplanting the "behavior modification" craze of the 1970s. The set point concept pervades both scientific and lay literature, but exactly what is it, where does it originate, what makes it so popular and how does this concept affect the management of obesity?

The body weight set point concept theorizes that the body is under a physiologic control system which "defends" and maintains a narrow range of weight or level of adiposity. The origin of this concept has its basis in the feedback control models introduced by systems engineers. Set point regulators maintain variables in a physical system at fixed values and make necessary alterations in the system to defend those values when challenged. The principle is similar to a home thermostat set at a fixed temperature. Is body weight, like temperature, pH, blood glucose, etc., under some form of homeostatic control? Can a physiologic mechanism (weight regulation) be explained via a set point model? Research in this area has demonstrated that both laboratory animals [32,33] and man [6,34,35] are able to maintain body weight within a narrow range over long periods. Furthermore, individuals have been shown to vigorously defend a particular weight after a forced 25 percent weight reduction [36], or 15–25 percent weight increase [37]. Much of the research which supports the set point theory of body weight regulation has been with hypothalmic-lesioned rats. It has been shown that LH-lesioned rats will defend their body weight in much the same fashion as non-lesioned animals, but at a lower weight [38]. This pattern of weight defense occurs when dietary mainpulation renders the meal both highly palatable [39] and unpalatable [40]. On the other hand, VMH-lesioned rats do not display the normal pattern of body weight defense upon certain dietary manipulations. While inappropriate subjects for study in the set point concept, the VMH-lesioned rats serve as a model for the "finickiness syndrome" illustrated in the investigations of Schachter and his colleagues [41,42].

The Zucher fatty is a genetically predisposed obese strain of rats. Unlike the VMH-lesioned rat and similar to the LH-lesioned rat, the Zucher fatty will vigorously defend its body weight, even when confronted with a caloric dilution and unpalatable diets [5]. Because the Zucher fatty rat will defend an obese weight, it may be an appropriate model for studying obese humans with elevated numbers of fat cells.

Given that the set point theory has merit, what factors can be controlled in weight maintenance? Body weight is a function of the balance of kilocalories consumed over kilocalories expended. Which, if either, variable exerts a greater influence over weight regulation? Of importance in treating obesity is the knowledge that lower weights due to forced weight reduction will require fewer calories because of reduced metabolism. A drastic reduction in kilocalories from maintenance levels will result in a drop in O_2 consumption and energy expenditure—a metabolic response of lowered caloric need compensating for reduced caloric intake.

Keyes and his associates [36] demonstrated that during a 24 week period of semi-starvation, human subjects actually reached a state of energy balance. Initial weight loss was rapid, but by the end of the period weight remained stable. During this study it was found that the basal metabolic rate dropped approximately 29% from the prerestriction rate. After correction for the loss of metabolic tissue, basal rate was still 16% lower than the original levels. In an experiment by Bray [43], daily caloric intake of obese patients was dropped from 3,500 kilocalories to 450 kilocalories. Weight loss was minimal (less than 3%) and tapered off after the first several weeks. O_2 consumption declined more than 17% while on the low kilocalorie diet, indicating that a decrease in energy expenditure was greater than the loss of tissue. Thus, weight loss is inhibited by an increase in the efficiency of energy utilization resulting from a metabolic adaptation (Figure 1).

In a similar fashion, weight displacement was resisted when a subject consumed almost two times the number of kilocalories needed to maintain a usual weight of 139 pounds. Weight gain

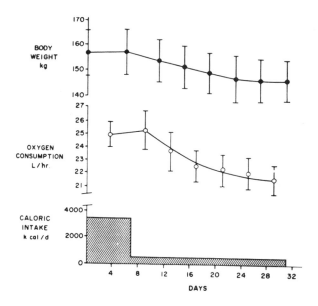

Figure 1. Effect of caloric intake on body-weight and energy expenditure of six obese patients. Caloric intake was reduced from 3500 to 450 C. on day 7. The point representing mean body-weight occur at the end of the 7th day and then every 4th day. Estimates of energy expenditure are the mean (± S.E.M.) of the measurements taken over the period bracketed by the data on body-weight and are placed at the midpoint of each period.

did not exceed 14%, even after weeks of an increased caloric consumption. Comparing the energy expenditure of LH-lesioned rats and normal rats indicates that caloric intake, in relation to tissue mass, is the same for both groups of animals. Energy expenditure is also normal. The lean LH-lesioned rat maintains a weight range in the same fashion as the non-lesioned rat, but at a lowered body weight. Conversely, when adjustments are calculated for the increase in metabolically active tissue, both the caloric intake and the energy expenditure of the Zucher fatty are maintained at rates similar to lean animals. Thus, the metabolic adaptations which occur in normal animals upon force feeding and caloric deprivation occur at much the same rate in lean LH-lesioned rats and Zucher fatty rats.

These data support the theory that weight is regulated around a body weight set point and that obese individuals may vigorously defend their weight at an elevated set point. If obese individuals lose weight through dieting, their basal metabolic rate decreases 15–30% with time. Bray [43] has shown that greater than a 20% reduction in metabolic rate can be reached in only two weeks. This rate decline, which begins 24–48 hours after initiating caloric restriction, is due to an increased efficiency of energy utilization and a decrease in energy expenditure [44]. Energy needs slowly drop in response to the lowered caloric consumption. Body weight then plateaus at the new obese weight despite the low calorie diet and if these individuals resume the previous caloric levels, a rapid weight gain occurs until the former level of obesity is reached.

The Effect of Physical Activity on Weight Control

Physical activity produces various metabolic consequences which enhance the weight loss process [45]. Exercise may facilitate weight loss by increasing the metabolic rate sufficiently to counter the drop in metabolic rate which occurs from dieting alone. Metabolic rate remains elevated for up to two hours after the cessation of exercise, indicating that the metabolic demands of exercise extend past the actual performance.

Lean body mass increases with exercise; thus, the proportion of metabolically active tissue gradually increases. Aerobic activity depends mainly on free fatty acids as its fuel source. Exercise enhances the mobilization and utilization of free fatty acids from adipose tissue, thus increasing fat weight loss and, at the same time, minimizes losses of lean mass [46]. Furthermore, exercise requires additional direct energy expenditure, raising the caloric need.

Physical activity has been shown to have a beneficial effect on yet another physiological process. Moderate amounts of vigorous exercise may actually decrease appetite, thus reducing caloric consumption. Although the appetite suppression resulting from exercise may be stronger in obese than in lean individuals, it will, in either case, reduce the caloric input from the diet.

The benefits of exercise in a weight control program stem from a higher metabolic rate and increased energy expenditure plus a suppression of appetite, resulting in a lower caloric intake.

DIETARY FACTORS AFFECTING FAT DEPOSITION

Dietary trends in modern societies have undergone some significant changes which have been correlated with an increased prevalence of obesity. Over the period between 1909 and 1980 in the U.S., a review of per capita food use [47] indicates increased consumption of meat, poultry, fish, dairy products, fats and oils, fruits, vegetables, sugars and other sweeteners, and decreasing intakes of eggs, potatoes, and grain products. The trend in food usage is reflected in the nutrient level of the diet. Kilocalories were slightly higher in 1980 than in 1909, but the proportion of kilocalories from fat increased 11%, while kilocalories from carbohydrates dropped 10%, with protein remaining the same. A significant alteration in the food supply is the 21% decrease in complex carbohydrates over this period and the reciprocal increase in simple carbohydrates owing to sugars and sweeteners added to foods. Similarly, a considerable change has evolved in the source of protein in the diet, although overall the level of protein has remained fairly constant. Whereas vegetable and animal proteins contributed equally to the food supply in 1909, animal products provided more than two-thirds of the total protein in 1980. These statistics are not surprising in light of the increased use of meats, poultry, fish, and dairy products, and the decline in the use of grain products. In 1980, beef alone contributed 16% of the protein intake compared to 19% from grain products.

A review by Scalfani [48] of the dietary factors affecting obesity heightens the significance of these data. Studies on laboratory animals indicate that when the percentage of kilo-calories as fat, which is 2–6% in standard chow, is raised to 30–60%, both the rates of weight gain and the fat deposition increase. High fat diets increase caloric intake and improve the efficiency of food utilization. Since fats are more than two times the caloric density of carbohydrate and protein, high fat diets provide more kilocalories than standard chow despite a lesser food intake. Fat stimulates appetite, increasing the palatability of the diet by improving both taste and texture of the food. Although rats ate less of the high fat diet, they consumed enough to increase caloric intake 10–20% over that of the standard chow. Rats fed a high fat diet deposit a greater proportion of energy as body fat than do rats fed a low fat chow. This seems to be due to an improved efficiency of food utilization attributed to the lower energy cost of converting dietary fat to body fat.

The concentration and type of dietary fat also affects food intake efficiency and food utilization of body weight [48]. Weight gain is enhanced by solid fats and long chain triglycerides rather than vegetable oils and short chain triglycerides. The degree to which these factors affect adiposity is influenced by age, sex, and strain of the animal. Obesity induced by a high fat diet is often reversible with a switch to a low fat diet, yet rats subsequently fed a high fat ration gained 40% more weight than rats previously fed chow. Exercise effectively reduces the degree of obesity in rats fed a high fat diet as long as the exercise is maintained.

Like high fat diets, but to a lesser degree, diets high in sugar promote obesity [48]. Compared to a starch diet, a high sucrose diet causes a greater fat deposition as a result of a sucrose-induced enhancement in the intestinal transport of sugar and an elevation in serum insulin levels. Sucrose in solution as a supplement to a chow diet proves to exert a stronger effect than a high sucrose diet. Although with a sucrose solution rats decrease their chow intake, they do not decrease it sufficiently to compensate for the additional kilocalories in the supplement. The palatability of the sucrose solution is a factor which stimulates appetite.

An interesting experiment with dietary manipulation studied the effect of a supermarket diet. Scalfani and Springer [49] offered adult rats chocolate chip cookies, salami, cheese, bananas, marshmallows, milk chocolate, peanut butter, and sweetened condensed milk, in addition to their chow, and observed a 269% greater weight gain than in rats fed only chow. Other experiments with supermarket foods have shown similar results. Supermarket foods may also cause adipocyte hyperplasia, thus elevating body weight even after a return to chow diets.

SOCIAL/ENVIRONMENTAL FACTORS INFLUENCING WEIGHT

Social environment is inextricably linked to the makeup of an individual. The effects, either positive or negative, of that environment are factors to be considered and addressed in any weight control program. When faced with a strongly negative social environment, the patient is not likely to continue weight management techniques. Patients can be taught to control their own behavior, but such change does not necessarily control the behavior of others. "Environmental sabotage," consciously or unconsciously executed, is a forceful influence few people are able to overcome.* Many of the behavioral techniques aimed at weight reduction require the cooperation and assistance of "significant others." For some patients this support is a readily available resource, waiting only to be trained and tapped. For others, there is indifference, fear, even resentment and hostility within the social environment.

*See P. Hodgson, Environmental sabotage: social, physical, and mental factors. In *Behavioral Management of Obesity* (New York, Spectrum Publications, 1984).

Outside the immediate environment of family and friends is the work world and the "cultural world." The cultural world refers to the culture in which we live and how it directly effects us in an impersonal way, for instance, the influence of television, magazines, newspapers, advertisements, restaurants, amusement parks, and recreational activities. As an example of the influence restaurants can have on one's attempt to lose weight, consider the patient who, for one reason or another, eats in restaurants the majority of the time. His ability to control his food intake is confined to the limits of the menu. The subliminal effect of the power of suggestion in food advertisements found in magazines, newspapers, and television is another powerful force of the "cultural world."

In the work world, patients are faced with morning doughnuts or Danish and coffee, business lunches, dinner meetings, and, of course, the "drink"—at lunch, after work, with dinner. As any good host knows, you must indulge and imbibe so your client feels "free" to have his or her fill.

In our rushed and harried society, we look to speed and convenience in eating. Prepackaged, precooked, prepared foods often comprise a significant portion of a patient's diet. Recent statistics indicate that one out of every three food dollars is spent in restaurants. When things get particularly rushed or when you simply "deserve a break," fast foods often fill the bill. Families in which both husband and wife work outside the home, single working parents, and individuals living alone tend to rely on time- and effort-saving convenience foods. Strained economic conditions cause people to adjust eating behaviors within a limited budget.

Often, a stigma is attached to being overweight and once stigmatization has occurred, the individual attaches a negative connotation to weight. Discussing the social consequences of obesity, Tobias and Gordon [50] caution against "a pat weight-reducing or control plan" and advise establishing short and long term goals. Identifying individual eating habits and nutritional peculiarities and understanding the physiologic ramifications of such are crucial to weight control. An appreciation of the whys and wherefores of nutritional modification will often provide additional motivation for making appropriate food selection.

Initially, and even recently, it was believed by some that dietary manipulation alone would suffice to cause weight loss. In fact, earlier investigations reported significant fat losses resulting from fasting and a ketogenic diet [51]. Other studies [52] utilizing very low calorie diets report losses of protein and water in addition to fat. A review of the literature [53], however, indicates that optimal body compostion changes are a result of a balanced diet of moderate caloric restriction plus regular aerobic exercise of sufficient duration and intensity. The incorporation of exercise into the program not only physiologically enhances weight loss but psychologically fosters positive eating behaviors. [For further discussion of the behavioral aspects of weight control refer to *Behavioral Management of Obesity* (New York, Spectrum Publications, 1984.)]

Weight loss and maintenance of weight loss should not be the only goals of a weight management program [53]. Eating a more nutritious diet, increasing activity, and possibly acceptance of current weight may be most realistic for some individuals.

SUMMARY

Body weight, the end product of energy balance, is influenced by numerous factors. Genetic endowment may predispose an individual toward leanness or fatness, yet social and environmental forces may override genetic tendencies. A popular theory is the set point concept of weight regulation which states that the body will maintain a weight or level of adiposity within a narrow range.

Even if this theory is proven to be true, there are yet other factors which govern weight. Parts of the social/environmental milieu are eating habits, nutritional composition of the diet, and exercise behaviors. These social/environmental factors strongly influence not only what we do but why and how often we do it. In short, people and culture can exert a positive or negative persuasion on eating and exercise behaviors, and cannot be ignored when designing a weight control program. Restricting calories alone may not be sufficient to tip the energy scale and induce a weight loss. We have come to recognize that increased proportions of calories as fat and simple carbohydrates (1) enhance palatability of the diet, (2) increase appetite, (3) improve the efficiency of energy utilization, and (4) raise calories due to the caloric concentration.

Thirty minutes or more of aerobic exercise 4–6 times per week aids in weight control from two vantage points. Physiologically, increased activity (1) raises caloric expenditure, (2) dulls appetite, (3) mobilizes free fatty acids from fat depots, and (4) combats a decline in basal metabolism associated with caloric restriction. Psychologically, regular exercise reinforces the concept of wellness—of doing something positive for health—and it provides an outlet for stress which may otherwise lead to inappropriate eating behaviors.

When developing and guiding clients through a weight control program, the counselor is wise to consider all factors which effect the regulation of energy balance. In doing so, the plan, as well as the goals, of such a program will be more realistic and achievable.

REFERENCES

1. Keys, A., and Brozek, J. Body fat in adult man. *Physiol. Rev. 33*: 245-325, 1953.
2. Stunkard, A. M. (ed.) *Obesity.* Philadelphia, W. B. Saunders Co., 1980.
3. Brody, S. *Bioenergetics and Growth.* New York, Reinhold Publishing Corp., p. 12, 1945.
4. Foch, T. T., and McClearn, G. E. Genetics, Body Weight and Obesity. In A. S. Stunkard (ed.), *Obesity.* Philadelphia, W. B. Saunders, 1980.
5. Cruce, J. A. F., Greenwood, J. R. C., Johnson, P. R., et al. Genetics versus hypothalmic obesity: studies of intake and dietary manipulation. *J. Comp. Physiol. Psychol. 97*:295-301, 1974.
6. *Ten-State Nutrition Survey,* 1968-1970. U.S. DHEW, Publication No. (HSM) 72-8131.
7. Garn, S., and Clark, D. C. Nutrition growth development and maturation: findings from the Ten-State Nutrition Survey of 1968-1970. *Pediatrics 56*:306-319, 1975.

8. Mayer, J. Decreased activity and energy balance in the hereditary obesity-diabetes syndrome of mice, *Science 117*:504-505, 1953.
9. Teitelbaum, P. Disturbances in feeding and drinking behavior after hypothalmic lesions. In M. A. Jones (ed.), *Nebraska Symposium on Motivation.* Lincoln Nebraska, University of Nebraska Press, 1961.
10. Hoebel, B. G., and Teitelbaum, P. Weight regulation in normal and hypothalmic hyperphagic rats. *J. Comp. Physiol. Psychol. 61*:189-193, 1976.
11. Frohman, A. L., and Bernadis, L. L. Effect of hypothalmic stimulation on plasma glucose, insulin and glucagon levels. *Amer. J. Physiol. 221*:1596-1603, 1971.
12. Bray, G. A. *The Obese Patient,* Philadelphia, W. B. Saunders Co., 1976.
13. Friedman, M. I. Effects of alloran diabetes on hypothalmic hyperphagia and obesity. *Amer. J. Physiol. 222*:174-178, 1972.
14. Hernandez, L., and Hoebel, B. G. Basic mechanism of feeding and weight regulation. In A. S. Stunkard (ed.), *Obesity.* Philadelphia, W. B. Saunders Co., 1980.
15. Ellison, G. D., and Sorenson, C. A. Two feeding syndromes following surgical isolation of the hypothalmus in rats. *J. Comp. Physiol. Psychol. 70*:173-188, 1970.
16. Kennedy, G. C. The role of depot fat in the hypothalmic control of food intake in the rat. *Proc. Royal Soc. J. 140*:578-592, 1953.
17. Liebelt, R. A., Ichinae, S., and Nicholson, N. Regulatory influences of adipose tissue on food intake and body weight. *Ann. N.Y. Academy Sci. 131*:559-582, 1965.
18. McCane, R. Food, Growth and Time. *Lancet 2*:671-676, 1962.
19. Faust, I. M., Johnson, P. R., and Hirsch, J. Noncompensation of adipose mass in partially lipectomized mice or rats. *Amer. J. Physiol. 231*:538-544, 1976.
20. Kral, J. Surgical reduction of adipose tissue in the male Sprague-Dawley rat. Effects on body composition, adipose tissue cellularity and lipid and carbohydrate metabolism. *Amer. J. Physiol. 231*:1090, 1976.
21. Hirsch, J., and Knittle, J. L. Cellularity of obese and non-obese human adipose tissue. *Fed. Proc. 29*:1516-1521, 1970.
22. Hager, A., Sjostrom, L., Arvidsson, B., et al. Body fat and adipose tissue cellularity in infants: a longitudinal study. *Metab. 26*:607-614, 1977.
23. Sjöström, L. Fat cells and body weight. In A. S. Stunkard (ed.), *Obesity.* Philadelphia, W. B. Saunders Co., 1980.

24. Faust, I. M., Johnson, P., Stern, J., et al. Diet-induced adipocyte number increase in adult rats: a new model of obesity. *Amer. J. Physiol. 235*:E 299-E 286, 1978.
25. Johnson, P. R., Stern, J., Gruen, R., et al. Development of adipose depot cellularity, plasma insulin, pancreatic insulin release and insulin resistance in the Zucker obese female rat. *Fed. Proc. 35*:657, 1976.
26. Bjorntrop, P., and Sjostrom, L. Number and size of adipose tissue fat cells in relation to metabolism in human obesity. *Metabolism 20*:703-713, 1971.
27. Hirsch, J., and Batchelor, B. Adipose cellularity in human obesity. *Clinics in Endocrinol. Metab. 5*:299-311, 1976.
28. Sjostrom, L., and Bjorntrop, P. Body composition and adipose tissue cellularity in human obesity. *Acta Med. Scand. 195*:201-211, 1974.
29. Bjorntrop, P., Gustafson, A., and Persson, B. Adipose tissue fat cell size and number in relation to metabolism in endogenous hypertriglyceridemia, *Acta Med. Scand. 190*:363-367, 1971.
30. Matter, S., et al. Body fat content and serum lipid levels. *J. Amer. Diet. Assoc. 77*:149-152, 1980.
31. Krotkiewski, M., Sjostrom, L., Bjorntrop, P., et al. Adipose tissue cellularity in relation to prognosis for weight reduction. *Internatl. J. Obesity 1*:395-416, 1977.
32. Brooks, C., and Lambert, E. F. A study of the effect of limitation of food intake and the method of feeding on the rate of weight gain during hypothalmic obesity in the albino rat. *Amer. J. Physiol. 147*: 695-707, 1946.
33. Cohn, C., and Joseph, D. Influence of body weight and body fat on appetite of "Normal" lean and obese rats. *Yale J. Biol. Med. 34*: 598-607, 1962.
34. Khosha, T., Billewicz, W. Z. Measurement of changes in body weight. *Brit. J. Nutr. 18*:227-239, 1964.
35. Robinson, M. D., and Watson, P. E. Day to day variation in body weight of young women. *Brit. J. Nutr. 19*:225-235, 1965.
36. Keyes, A., Brozek, J., Henschel, A., et al. *The Biology of Human Starvation.* Minneapolis, University of Minnesota Press, 1958.
37. Sims, E. A., and Horton, E. S. Endocrin and metabolic adaptation of obesity and starvation. *Amer. J. Clin. Nutr. 21*:1455-1470, 1968.
38. Mitchel, J. S., and Keesey, R. E. Defense of a lowered body weight maintenance level by lateral hypothalamically lesioned rats: evidence from a restriction-feeding regimen. *Physiol. Behavior 18*:1121-1125, 1977.

39. Powley, T. L., and Keesey, R. E. Relationship of body weight to the lateral hypothalmic feeding syndrome. *J. Comp. Physiol.* 70:25–36, 1970.
40. Keesey, R. E., and Boyle, P. C. Effects of quinine adulteration upon body weight of LH-lesioned and intact male rat. *J. Comp. Physiol. Psychol.* 84:38–46, 1973.
41. Nisbitt, R. E. Hunger, obesity and the ventromedial hypothalmus. *Psychol. Rev.* 79:433–453, 1972.
42. Schacter, S. Some extraordinary facts about obese humans and rats. *Amer. Psychol.* 26:129–144, 1971.
43. Bray, G. A. Effect of caloric restriction on energy expenditure in obese patients. *Lancet* 2:397–398, 1969.
44. Apfelbaum, M., Bostsarron, J., and Lacatis, D. Effect of caloric restriction and excessive caloric intake on energy expenditure. *Amer. J. Clin. Nutr.* 24:1405–1409, 1971.
45. Brownell, K. D., and Stunkard, A. J. Physical activity in the development and control of obesity. In A. J. Stunkard (ed.) *Obesity.* Philadelphia, W. B. Saunders, 1980.
46. McArdle, W. D., Katch, F. I., and Katch, V. L. *Exercise Physiology.* Philadelphia, Lea and Febiger, 1981.
47. Welsch, S., and Martson, R. M. Review of trends in food use in the U.S., 1909–1980. *J. Amer. Diet. Assoc.* 81:120–125, 1980.
48. Scalfani, A. Dietary Obesity. In A. J. Stunkard (ed.), *Obesity.* Philadelphia, W. B. Saunders, 1980.
49. Scalfani, A., and Springer, D. Dietary obesity in adult rats: similarities to hypothalmic and human obesity syndromes. *Physiol. Behavior 17:* 461–471, 1976.
50. Tobias, A. L., and Gordon, J. B. "Social Consequences of Obesity." *J. Am. Dietet. Assoc.* 76:338–342, 1980.
51. Benoit, F. L., Martin, R. L., and Watters, R. H. Changes in body composition during weight reduction in obesity. *Ann. Inter. Medicine 63* (4):604–612, 1965.
52. Passmore, R., Strong, J. A., and Ritchie, F. J. The chemical composition of the tissue lost by obese patients in a reducing regimen, *Br. J. Nutr.* 12:113–122, 1958.
53. American College of Sports Medicine. Position statement on proper and improper weight loss programs. *Med. Sci. in Sports and Exercise 15*:ix–xiii, 1983.

3

Medical Indications for Weight Reduction

Charles P. Lucas

INTRODUCTION

Men and women who are above average weight have an increased likelihood of dying at a younger age than people of average weight. Table 1, taken from the 1979 Build and Blood Pressure Study of the Society of Actuaries [1], describes this relationship, constructed from data on nearly 100,000 insured deaths. Men in the bracket 15% below to 5% above average weight have a relative risk less than the population average of 100. Between 15-25% above average weight, the risk for men is 117, rising to 186 when weight is 55-65% above average. For women who weigh 15% below to 5% above average, the risk is also less than 100, while in the group 45-55% above average

Copyright © 1984 by Spectrum Publications, Inc., *Evaluation and Treatment of Obesity*, edited by J. Storlie and H. A. Jordan.

Table 1. Mortality Ratios in Men and Women in Various Categories of Weight Compared to Average[a]

Percent departure from average weight	Ratio of actual to Expected mortality × 100	
	Men	Women
25–35% Underweight	117	128
15–25% Underweight	102	111
5–15% Underweight	95	93
Within 5% of average	95	97
5–15% Overweight	106	100
15–25% Overweight	117	109
25–35% Overweight	130	103
35–45% Overweight	139	109
45–55% Overweight	168	131
55–65% Overweight	186	140

[a] Adapted from table in Reference 1, p. 52, 1979 Build and Blood Pressure Study of the Society of Actuaries, with permission.

weight, the risk increases to 130. These data thus indicate that men are more adversely affected by obesity than women.

Table 1 reveals the fact that persons of below average weight also died at a younger age, a finding in agreement with results obtained from the Framingham study [2], where a U- or J-shaped mortality curve describes the relationship between relative weight and mortality, and is at variance with the Build and Blood Pressure Study of 1959 [3], which failed to find increased mortality at the low end of the weight curve. In the Framingham study the increased number of deaths in leaner individuals occurred in a group where tobacco use was high. Eighty percent of this group of below average weight individuals were cigarette smokers, 1.6 times the population average. Nevertheless, not all of this excess mortality could be explained on the use of tobacco. Indeed, deaths in the very lean are likely to occur for a variety of reasons [1]. Underweight men in the Build and Blood Pressure Study died more often of malignant neoplasms (130% of average), hypertensive heart disease (130% of average), pneumonia and influenza (160% of average),

Table 2. Average Weights of Men. Graduated Weights (in Indoor Clothing) in Pounds[a]

Height (in shoes)	Age Groups							
	15–16	17–19	20–24	25–29	30–39	40–49	50–59	60–69
4'10"	93	106	112	116	120	121	122	121
11"	98	110	117	121	124	126	127	126
5'0"	102	115	121	125	129	131	132	130
1"	107	119	126	130	133	135	136	135
2"	112	124	130	134	138	140	141	140
3"	116	129	136	140	143	144	145	144
4"	121	132	139	143	147	149	150	149
5"	127	137	143	147	151	154	155	153
6"	133	141	148	152	156	158	159	158
7"	137	145	153	156	160	163	164	163
8"	143	150	157	161	165	167	168	167
9"	148	155	163	166	170	172	173	172
10"	153	159	167	171	174	176	177	176
11"	159	164	171	175	179	181	182	181
6'0"	162	168	176	181	184	186	187	186
1"	168	174	182	186	190	192	193	191
2"	173	179	187	191	195	197	198	196
3"	178	185	193	197	201	203	204	200
4"	184	190	198	202	206	208	209	207
5"	189	195	203	207	211	213	214	212
6"	195	201	209	213	217	219	220	218
7"	201	207	215	219	223	225	226	224

[a] Adapted from Table 24, p. 39, 1979 Build and Blood Pressure Study of the Society of Actuaries, with permission.

Table 3. Average Weights of Women. Graduated Weights (in Indoor Clothing) in Pounds[a]

Height (in shoes)	Age Groups							
	15–16	17–19	20–24	25–29	30–39	40–49	50–59	60–69
4'6"	85	87	89	95	101	105	109	111
7"	89	91	93	98	104	108	112	114
8"	93	95	99	103	107	111	115	117
9"	97	99	101	106	110	114	118	120
10"	101	103	105	110	113	118	121	123
11"	105	108	110	112	115	121	125	127
5'0"	109	111	112	114	118	123	127	130
1"	112	115	116	119	121	127	131	133
2"	117	119	120	121	124	129	133	136
3"	121	123	124	125	128	133	137	140
4"	123	126	127	128	131	136	141	143
5"	128	129	130	132	134	139	144	147
6"	131	132	133	134	137	143	147	150
7"	135	136	137	138	141	147	152	155
8"	138	140	141	142	145	150	156	158
9"	142	145	146	148	150	155	159	161
10"	146	148	149	150	153	158	162	163
11"	149	150	155	156	159	162	166	167
6'0"	152	154	157	159	164	168	171	172
1"	155	157	159	163	168	172	175	176
2"	158	160	162	166	172	176	179	180
3"	161	163	165	170	176	180	183	184

[a] Adapted from Table 25, p. 40, 1979 Build and Blood Pressure Study of the Society of Actuaries, with permission.

diseases of the digestive system (140% of average), and suicides (140% of average). On the other hand overweight individuals suffered greater mortality from diabetes (up to 500% of average), diseases of the heart and circulatory system (up to 200% of average), coronary artery disease (up to 180% of average), and vascular lesions of the central nervous system (130% of average).

It is now general medical knowledge that weight loss improves, and even reverses, such conditions as hypertension, diabetes and hyperlipidemia. Based on actuarial data, weight loss is associated with decreased mortality [3], and hygienically achieved weight reduction in obese individuals with these conditions is highly desirable. It is no surprise, therefore, that the discovery of newer modalities for the treatment of obesity has rekindled interest in its application to the treatment of these diseases. The Society of Actuaries, through the Build and Blood Pressure Study of 1979, has published tables of optimal weights which should serve as target weight guidelines (Tables 2 and 3). Based on these data it is recommended that weight be maintained at average or near average weight for age and height, although each individual case should be judged on the risks and benefits involved.

CAUSE OF DEATH IN OBESITY

Heart disease is clearly the most common cause of death in very obese individuals, yet there is little consensus and incomplete understanding of the role obesity plays in its development. Epidemiological evidence, for example, suggests a weak relationship between obesity and cardiovascular disease [4,5]. However, these studies of middle age American males share a variety of defects. The populations studied were generally 20 to 25% above ideal weight, had few lean individuals, and many cigarette smokers in the far leaner samples. Given these general features, it has been difficult to make appropriate comparisons of obesity related morbidity and mortality. In Hawaii, where a more heterogenous group of Japanese males have been studied, markedly lower risk was found in leaner subjects [6]. More recently data has been reported from a Framingham population where a larger proportion of young, leaner individuals provided a better opportunity to study the effect of obesity on both serum cholesterol and its lipoprotein carriers [7]. In a group of 20–29 year old males, still containing many lean individuals, 50% of those whose relative body weight was greater than 140% had a ratio in serum of total to HDL cholesterol greater than 5.0. On the other hand, in those whose relative body weight was equal to or less than 100%, the ratio of total to HDL cholesterol in serum was greater than 5.0 in only 5% of the sample. For this ratio to be high (5 and above) in obese individuals, is relevant because subjects with elevated ratios of total to HDL cholesterol in serum suffer higher morbidity and mortality from coronary artery disease [8]. Because obesity appears to also increase the likelihood of hypertension and diabetes mellitus, it is not unreasonable to assume, therefore, that obesity causes cardiovascular disease because of its strong association with all of these known cardiovascular risk factors.

WEIGHT LOSS IN THE MANAGEMENT OF TYPE II DIABETES MELLITUS OR NON-INSULIN DEPENDENT DIABETES MELLITUS (NIDDM)

It is estimated that the most common form of diabetes mellitus today is what was formerly called adult-onset diabetes mellitus, now referred to as Type II diabetes mellitus or non-insulin dependent diabetes mellitus (NIDDM). NIDDM is characteristically associated with obesity in 80% of cases, and with insulin resistance in almost all instances [9]. This section reviews the pathophysiology of NIDDM, and the effectiveness of its treatment with weight loss and diet.

Insulin Secretion in NIDDM

DeFronzo has recently reviewed the role of insulin secretion in NIDDM. Based on data from 47 studies [9], he concluded that the insulin response to a glucose load was deficient in most patients with fasting hyperglycemia, and that when the fasting plasma glucose exceeds 160-180 mg/dl, the plasma insulin response to glucose is quite flat.

In chemical diabetes, now called impaired glucose tolerance, where fasting blood glucose concentration is in the normal range, the situation is quite variable. Most investigators report normal or even increased insulin response to glucose in chemical diabetes. If this is so, what then causes a progression of disease from chemical diabetes to overt diabetes mellitus with fasting hyperglycemia in a significant percentage of patients [10]? The most likely explanation is found in the work of a number of investigators, beginning with Himsworth [11], who have demonstrated that patients with NIDDM characteristically have insulin resistance [12-17], and that this abnormality in insulin resistance is accompanied by an inherent "defect" in pancreatic synthesis and/or release of insulin [18].

Insulin Resistance in NIDDM

Impaired insulin action, or insulin resistance, in NIDDM has been studied in individuals of normal weight, in order to differentiate it from the insulin resistance which is also typical of obese non-diabetic subjects [19,20]. Indeed the obese subject with normal glucose tolerance shares the same abnormalities as the normal weight NIDDM patient with respect to the site of insulin action in liver and peripheral tissues, and in the cellular location of resistance, i.e., the receptor and post-receptor defect. Since most patients with NIDDM are also obese, this defect in insulin resistance is commonly a summation of these two forces. A third important contributing factor is the relative physical inactivity of the majority of NIDDM patients who would benefit from the improved insulin action of exercise [21,22].

The impaired insulin action in NIDDM is accompanied by decreased insulin mediated glucose disposal in peripheral insulin-sensitive tissues like muscle and fat [23], and also by subnormal suppression of hepatic glucose output [24]. The mechanism of insulin resistance in NIDDM is due to impairment of insulin action on target cells. Two categories of insulin resistance have been identified: (a) that due to decreased insulin binding to cellular receptors as a consequence of reduced numbers of receptors [25,26], and (b) that due to defective effector system(s) in cells beyond the receptor, the so-called "post-receptor defect" [25,26]. In patients with mildly impaired glucose tolerance, the degree of post-receptor defect is minimal and insulin resistance correlates significantly with a reduction in insulin receptors observed on isolated monocytes [25,26]. In more severe degrees of NIDDM, evidenced by significant fasting hyperglycemia (200 mg/dl), the degree of post-receptor defect, as well as net insulin resistance, is more marked, and a poor correlation exists between net insulin resistance and receptor numbers on isolated monocytes [25,26].

Thus, where there is more severe hypoinsulinemia, there is more severe insulin resistance or less insulin action. Scarlett et al. [27] tested the hypothesis that the marked insulin resistance of more advanced NIDDM was due to insulin deficiency, or hyperglycemia, or both. They utilized aggressive, short-term insulin therapy to maintain blood glucose in the range of 100 mg/dl (mean blood glucose 114 mg/dl) for a 14 day period of time. At the end of this period of intensive insulin therapy, they observed that insulin sensitivity, measured by the glucose clamp techique, improved toward that of normal subjects. The primary improvement in insulin action was a decrease in resistance associated with the post-receptor defect. In summary, the pathophysiology of NIDDM is characterized by hypoinsulinemia and insulin resistance, the latter due, early on, to less insulin receptors, and later to a combination of a receptor and post-receptor defect(s), that can be reversed by correction of blood glucose with insulin.

Treatment of NIDDM

Insulin. Treatment of the obese patient with NIDDM can be approached by attacking the pathophysiologic hallmarks of the disease: insulin insufficiency and/or insulin resistance. Scarlett et al. [27] were able to demonstrate that intensive insulin therapy not only corrected the insulin insufficiency (and the hyperglycemia) but also made a significant impact on the accompanying insulin resistance. Indeed, insulin therapy is necessary when marked hyperglycemia is present, especially under conditions of stress, illness, or surgery. In the majority of instances, however, insulin treatment as it is currently used does no more than barely control the hyperglycemia (usually in the 150–250% mg/dl range). Under these circumstances insulin therapy does little to alleviate the underlying pathophysiologic abnormalities of NIDDM. Indeed, it often leads to further weight gain, and thus, more insulin resistance.

Nonpharmacologic Treatment—Diet. Dietary treatment offers a better alternative for the treatment of NIDDM because of its ability to correct the pathophysiology which produced the diabetic state. Savage showed, for example, that correction of hyperglycemia was associated with a significant improvement in insulin secretion in six type II Pima Indian diabetics who lost 11 kg on a 500 calorie weight reduction diet [28]. Also observed was an improvement in binding of insulin to its cellular receptors. Utilizing a 300 calorie, 40 gram protein, 35 gram carbohydrate diet, Genuth, Vertes, and Hazelton have shown that patients with NIDDM, even if taking over 50 units of insulin per day, commonly attained normal, or nearly normal, fasting blood glucose values after 1–2 weeks of diet therapy [29]. The question raised from these findings is whether it is weight loss or carbohydrate restriction that leads to this improvement in blood glucose and insulin release. There is no question, from the timing of the response that carbohydrate restriction itself plays an improtant role. Carbohydrate excess, especially if it is predominantly sucrose or glucose aggravates fasting hyperglycemia in NIDDM [30], while low carbohydrate diets improve glucose tolerance even without weight loss [31]. On the other hand, the simple sugars fructose and sorbitol have a small effect on blood glucose and insulin secretion [32,33,34]. In addition, foods that contain complex carbohydrates are preferable to simple sugars like glucose and sucrose in treating patients with NIDDM, and some starches produce less hyperglycemia and hyperinsulinemia than others [33]. Indeed, diets high in carbohydrates but also high in fiber have a beneficial effect on blood glucose and insulin secretion [35,36].

A second advantage of dietary therapy results from its effect on weight. Weight loss, on a long-term basis, is capable of decreasing the fasting plasma glucose concentration, improving glucose tolerance, enhancing tissue sensitivity to insulin and improving insulin secretion [37–45]. Thus dietary therapy improves the pathophysiologic deficiencies of NIDDM, namely insulin insufficiency and insulin resistance. On the other hand, Savage et al. found that it may take several months for endogenous insulin secretion to return to normal, based on six months of dietary treatment of one Pima Indian diabetic patient [46].

Nonpharmacologic Treatment–Exercise. Weight loss is also likely to increase the patient's ability to exercise, especially if the weight loss program stresses exercise as an important treatment component. There are two favorable effects of exercise on glucose disposal; (a) that which occurs acutely in trained or untrained subjects, and (b) that which is observed in trained individuals. Commensurate with the onset of exercise, plasma insulin declines while blood levels of glucagon and catecholamines increase [47–51]. This fall in insulin and rise in glucagon and catecholamines favors enhanced release of free fatty acids (FFA) that supply working muscles with substrate. Short term exercise, whether performed by trained or untrained individuals, leads to marked stimulation of glucose uptake by contracting muscles [52,53]. This increase in glucose uptake is dependent upon the presence of circulating insulin [54,55]. In the absence of insulin glucose uptake by exercising muscles is markedly inhibited.

DeFronzo et al. have shown [56] that by administering insulin to exercising normal subjects, glucose sensitivity was increased by nearly twice the amount obtained from exercise alone or insulin alone. Though insulin sensitivity markedly improves in insulin dependent diabetes mellitus as a result of short term exercise, no comparable studies have been published in patients with NIDDM.

The effect of long term training on glucose disposal and insulin sensitivity has only recently been studied. Trained athletes have normal or supernormal glucose tolerance, despite a much reduced insulin secretory response to glucose challenge [57,58]. These results strongly support the concept of enhanced insulin sensitivity in trained individuals. Physical training has been shown to decrease fasting plasma insulin concentration, as well as glucose-stimulated insulin secretion in normal subjects and those with chemical diabetes with no overall change in glucose tolerance [59,60]. Soman et al. [61] showed that a six week training program, instituted in six healthy subjects, enhanced insulin sensitivity commensurate with an increase in VO_2 max. DeFronzo made a similar observation in six subjects with NIDDM [9].

In summary, weight loss offers a variety of theoretical advantages over insulin therapy and other non-reducing dietary treatments in NIDDM. A weight loss diet restricted in simple carbohydrates acutely corrects hyperglycemia, and over time improves insulin secretion, increases the concentration of insulin receptors and improves sensitivity to insulin. If it improves the patient's ability to exercise then an additional benefit is further enhancement of insulin sensitivity through the muscles' ability to utilize glucose. Oral hypoglycemic agents have not been considered in this discussion. Nevertheless, they offer theoretical and practical advantages in those patients whose blood glucose cannot be controlled to normal with weight loss and dietary therapy [62]. Figure 1 summarizes the foregoing discussion and describes the progression, and possible regression, of NIDDM. It describes how normal glucose tolerance can, under the influence of genetic and environmental factors, progress to overt fasting hyperglycemia. These environmental factors of excessive simple carbohydrate calories, physical inactivity, and resultant obesity continue to perpetuate and worsen the hyperglycemia by increasing insulin resistance even further. The fasting hyperglycemia acts, in some way, to abolish the pancreatic response to glucose loads, aggravating an already compromised system. Reversal of this process can be accomplished by exercise and dietary restriction of simple carbohydrates to correct the hyperglycemia rather

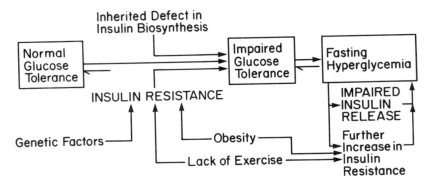

Figure 1. Progression and regression of noninsulin-dependent diabetes mellitis.

abruptly. Weight loss resolves the long term situation by improving insulin sensitivity. Although remission of NIDDM is theoretically possible, adequate reversal of environmental factors is infrequently accomplished to make this a common occurrence. It nevertheless should be every practitioner's goal for his patients.

WEIGHT REDUCTION FOR THE TREATMENT OF HYPERCHOLESTEROLEMIA

The effect of weight loss on levels of serum cholesterol is complex. Friedman et al. found that a 25 kg loss in weight resulted in a mean increase in serum HDL cholesterol of 8 mg/dl in a group of 15 women [63]. Schrott et al. on the other hand, found no significant change in serum HDL cholesterol concentration six months after gastric bypass surgery, when subjects (29 women and 9 men) had lost an average of 33 kg [64]. Indeed, average serum HDL cholesterol decreased by 8 mg/dl, while the average of total serum cholesterol also decreased from 198 to 176 mg/dl. The ratio of total to HDL cholesterol remained unchanged (4.7 to 4.8). Thompson et al. studied 15 obese females before and after eight months of behavior modification treatment for weight reduction [65]. An average of 12 kg of weight was lost. After eight weeks of weight reduction, they observed a small decrease in mean serum HDL cholesterol, which returned to baseline by eight months of follow-up. Multiple regression analysis indicated that in their study serum HDL cholesterol decreased during periods of rapid weight reduction. Brownell et al., also using behavior modification to produce weight loss, studied 73 obese men and women who lost an average of 10.7 and 8.9 kg, respectively [66]. In men, mean serum HDL cholesterol levels increased by 5% while mean serum LDL cholesterol decreased. In women, mean HDL cholesterol decreased slightly. Lucas et al. (unpublished data) have studied a total of 20 women who lost an average of 59 pounds using modified fasting and behavior modification. Mean total serum cholesterol, measured before and after weight loss, and, at a time when stable weight was attained, declined from 221 mg/dl to 209 mg/dl; mean serum HDL cholesterol levels rose from 52.8 to 57.6 mg/dl. Thus, the ratio of total to HDL cholesterol in serum declined from 4.18 to 3.63. Eight men who lost an average of 80 pounds were studied under similar circumstances. Mean total serum cholesterol decreased from 218 to 188 mg/dl, while mean serum HDL cholesterol remained the same (40.8 to 40.0). Thus, the ratio of total to HDL cholesterol declined from 5.34 to 4.70. Streja et al. studied 13 grossly obese patients (10 females, 3 males), who lost an average of 16.1 kg using a protein-modified fast [67]. The serum levels of total and HDL cholesterol were measured both before and six months after attainment of stable weight. Changes in total cholesterol and LDL cholesterol were not significant. However, the mean level of HDL cholesterol in serum increased significantly by 6 mg/dl, a change that inversely correlated with the amount of weight loss. The intercept of the regression relating serum HDL cholesterol of percentage change in weight was −7.3, indicating that a weight loss of at least 7.3% of body weight had to occur before an increase in serum HDL cholesterol could be observed.

In general, these data indicate that serum HDL cholesterol increases with weight loss while the ratio of total to HDL cholesterol decreases. A number of factors need to be considered in interpreting the variations observed from study to study. To begin with, the presence of diabetes mellitus [68], the level of physical activity, and the use of alcohol [69], by the obese or formerly obese patient are all important to consider, because of the known effect of these factors on HDL cholesterol. The study of Thompson is particularly important because it indicates that serum HDL cholesterol declines when measured during rapid weight loss [65]. Thus, patients who have had gastric bypass surgery and who are continuing to lose weight may not demonstrate the same HDL cholesterol response as those who have lost weight and who are studied during a period of stable weight. Finally, the findings of Streja et al. have special significance because they suggest that considerable weight loss (7.3% of body weight) must occur before changes in HDL cholesterol are evident. Further studies controlling for all of these critical variables may provide the information necessary to explain the mechanism(s) responsible for the improvement noted in the various lipoprotein cholesterol fractions with weight loss.

Whether these changes in HDL cholesterol or in the ratio of total cholesterol to HDL cholesterol explain the beneficial effect on mortality that has been observed with weight loss [3] remains to be proven. It must be kept in mind that whatever benefit might result in serum lipids from weight loss, continued or further improvement will require changes in the content of the maintenance diet. Such a diet should be low in cholesterol and saturated fat, that is, restrictive in the consumption of meat, cheese, whole milk, sausage, and other foods that contain saturated fats and oils.

WEIGHT LOSS AND THE MANAGEMENT OF THE HYPERTENSIVE PATIENT

Epidemiological data implicate high sodium intake as a cause for hypertension [70]. Simply put, populations who ingest larger amounts of salt have a higher incidence of hypertension than those with low salt intake. Indeed, it is unusual to find hypertension in populations where sodium intake is less than 85 mEq/24 hours. It should be pointed out, however, that a consistent relationship within populations, between sodium intake and blood pressure, cannot be demonstrated unless those with a positive family history of hypertension are examined separately [71]. This latter observation suggests that there are those whose blood pressure is resistant to sodium ingestion, and another group whose blood pressure is sensitive to sodium in the diet. Sodium restriction and challenge studies have also demonstrated that sodium, in some individuals, is an important clinical factor in hypertension [72].

These data are consistent with studies conducted in rats [73]. It was Dahl who first observed that rats can be bred to develop hypertension when challenged with a high salt diet. While these observations offer evidence that the phenomenon of salt sensitivity applies to species other than Homosapiens, they also provide insight into the etiology of hypertension. Observations made in stroke-prone salt-sensitive hypertensive rats reveal that high sodium intake blocks reuptake of norepinephrine by noradrenaline-releasing nerve endings of both normal and salt-sensitive rats [74]. In the latter, however, this phenomenon leads to inappropriately elevated plasma levels of norepinephrine because of lack of inhibition of centrally-mediated sympathetic tone.

Although obese individuals eat more salt than non-obese individuals [75], there are no further data to explain the higher incidence of hypertension of obesity on increased dietary intake of salt. In fact, studies by Reisin et al. have shown that weight reduction of 9–10 kg leads to a significant fall in blood pressure, even in the presence of a high sodium intake [76]. It is important to note, however, that sodium balance tends to be negative during active weight reduction. Although this phenomenon has a variety of possible explanations, there nevertheless exists a state of sodium rejection by the kidney such that a high salt intake would fail to effect net positive sodium balance during weight loss. Indeed, it is likely that negative caloric balance leads to natriuresis irrespective of sodium intake, and thus one of the reasons for the effectiveness of weight loss in lowering blood pressure may relate to the accompanying loss of sodium from the body.

There are other metabolic consequences of adiposity which could shed light on the etiology of hypertension in obesity. Sowers has shown that obese individuals have higher serum levels of norepinephrine than controls [77]. In obese subjects undergoing weight reduction he described a decline in the mean level of serum norepinephrine that paralleled the mean fall in blood pressure [78]. When obese people remain on a hypocaloric diet for several weeks, one of the frequent physiological consequences of this hormonal change is the development of postural dizziness and hypotension. One likely explanation for this decline in noradrenaline during caloric deprivation is believed to be the body's adaptive response, namely its attempt to decrease caloric expenditure when there is less caloric intake. In this regard, another calorigenic hormone, serum triiodothyronine is also decreased during periods of caloric restriction [79].

While infused noradrenaline raises blood pressure because of its direct vasopressor effect on vascular smooth muscle, its hypertensinogenic effect in obesity may also be mediated by its sodium retaining properties. Both the infusion of norepinephrine and stimulation of renal sympathetic nerves are associated with renal-mediated sodium retention [80]. Thus, factors which increase the activity of the sympathetic nervous system may have effects on blood pressure by the direct action of norepinephrine on vascular smooth muscles or via the sympathetic nervous system's effect on sodium conservation. One such factor is the ingestion of glucose itself. Young et al. observed in normal subjects that glucose, when orally administered, raised plasma norepinephrine levels to a greater extent than that seen following ingestion of a control drink [81]. Also, Rowe et al. observed that when glucose was given to normal subjects in combination with insulin, an increase in blood pressure, heart rate, and blood levels or norepinephrine ensued [82]. It is of interest that insulin alone can increase transport in sodium across the toad skin [83], and produces sodium reabsorption in isolated dog and intact human kidneys [84]. Since obese individuals typically have high blood levels of insulin, the possibility exists that insulin itself may be responsible for sodium retention in overweight individuals. Thus, enhanced retention of sodium by insulin and norepinephrine, both of which are increased by overfeeding, could contribute to the development of hypertension in obesity. Consistent with this hypothesis is the fact that restriction of calories in obese individuals is associated with a fall in both serum insulin [85] and serum norepinephrine [77], coincident with a fall in blood pressure and an intense natriuresis which cannot be explained by a decrease in renin or aldosterone [86]. Additionally, infusion of insulin prevents the natriuresis of fasting [87], making it likely that the fall in serum insulin and noradrenaline which occurs with weight loss, may explain the natriuresis of weight reduction.

Thus, the obese individual is exposed to an interplay of both high salt intake and hormones, noradrenaline, and insulin, which are an adaptation to his obese state. This situation has the capability of producing a more positive sodium balance, a condition that can enhance the blood pressure reactivity to catecholamines, perhaps through the mechanism of diminished reuptake of norepinephrine. The increased levels of serum norepinephrine resulting from overeating would thus have a positive effect on blood pressure. Figure 2 describes the pathophysiologic sequence that accounts for the high incidence of hypertension in obesity. It explains how environmental factors (increased carbohydrate ingestion and obesity) operate to

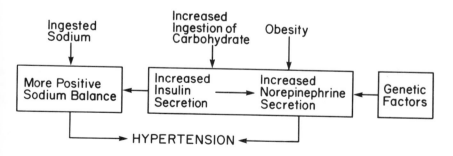

Figure 2. Sequence to explain high incidence of hypertension in obesity.

enhance insulin and norepinephrine secretion. The variation in response of obese subjects is probably under genetic control. The resultant effect is for insulin to enhance norepinephrine secretion, and for both of these hormones to enhance sodium retention. Under these circumstances norepinephrine causes more pronounced vasoconstriction and blood pressure elevation.

The role of exercise in this regard is important since exercise is known to decrease serum insulin [88] and the activity of the sympathetic nervous system [89]; these changes may explain its effect on lowering blood pressure. Krotkiewski et al. studied 27 obese women placed on a six month physical training program. Blood pressure decreased consistently after training. This fall was not correlated with weight loss, but was instead related to the initial concentration, and decrease of, serum insulin, glucose, and triglycerides [90].

The work of Geunth has shown that a hypocaloric diet used in the treatment of obesity can lead within one week to a correction of blood pressure to normal in two-thirds of hypertensive subjects [29]. A review of 21 studies on the effect of weight loss on blood pressure was made by Hovell, who concluded that blood pressure was significantly lowered by weight reduction [91]. The greatest effect of weight reduction on blood pressure occurs during the first week of dieting, during the period of intense natriuresis.

In summary, there is good circumstantial evidence that the hypertension of obesity is related to a combination of high salt and high caloric (carbohydrate) intake. The latter increases the levels of serum insulin in some individuals. The increased carbohydrate intake, either directly or via insulin, leads to a parallel increase in the level of noradrenaline; the blood pressure increases either from the direct effect of noradrenaline on vascular smooth muscle or via sodium retention, which potentiates the effect of noradrenaline on blood vessels. Low salt diet, weight reduction, exercise, and restriction of glucose should have a beneficial effect on blood pressure.

What kind of diet should be used? The diet must be sufficiently restricted in calories and be accompanied by behavior modification to permit reasonable success. During weight maintenance the diet should also be restricted in sugar and sodium. A diet containing less than 100 mEq of sodium is preferred. This can easily be obtained by encouraging the use of unprocessed meat or fish, low fat milk, fruits, fresh vegetables, and whole grains and cereals. Patients should be advised not to eat most cheeses (excluding low fat cottage cheese), and to avoid eating canned foods, processed meats, and certain condiments such as soy sauce, prepared mustards, ketchup, and seasoned salts. Fast food restaurants should also be avoided; indeed, great care must be taken in eating out.

Though the maintenance diet must be low in salt and restricted in calories to maintain weight, attention should be given also to its content of saturated fat, in view of recent evidence that a high polyunsaturated low-saturated fat diet lowered blood pressure even though salt intake was kept high [92].

Finally, considerable emphasis must be given to exercise in view of evidence that shows that it lowers blood pressure irrespective of weight loss. General exercises such as walking, running, swimming, or bicycling are encouraged.

SUMMARY AND CONCLUSION

It is hard to escape the fact that obesity predisposes people to coronary artery disease by its influence on blood sugar, lipoprotein metabolism, and blood pressure. It is also true that weight reduction, exercise, and long-term dietary restriction of calories, fats, and simple sugars can reverse these biochemical abnormalities which we call cardiovascular risk factors. Genetic influences probably explain why not all comparably obese people develop glucose intolerance, hypertension, or hypercholesterolemia. It is necessary, nevertheless, to consider the average obese person as one at higher than average risk, and to aggressively assess his or her degree of risk factor deviation, in order to provide the most complete prognosis for future health. Finally, the discussions in this chapter provide an updated view of the pathophysiologic sequences that lead to the development of these biochemical abnormalities, as well as a hopeful solution through aggressive intervention.

ACKNOWLEDGEMENT

The author is very greatful to Ms. Aulga Mahar for typing and helping with the manuscript.

REFERENCES

1. Build and Blood Pressure Study, 1979. Chicago, Society of Actuaries and Association of Life Insurance Medical Directors of America, pp. 1–255, 1980.
2. Sorlie, P., Gordon, T., and Kannel, W. B. Body Build and Mortality, The Framingham Study. *J.A.M.A. 243*:1828, 1980.
3. Build and Blood Pressure Study, 1959. Chicago, Society of Actuaries and Association of Life Insurance Medical Directors of America, pp. 1–268, 1959.
4. Kleinbaum, D. G., Kupper, L. L., Cassel, J. C., et al. Multi-variate analysis of risk of coronary artery disease in Evans County, Georgia. *Arch. Intern. Med. 128*:943, 1971.
5. Paul, O., Lepper, M. H., Phelaw, W. H., et al. A longitudinal study of coronary heart disease. *Circulation 28*:10, 1963.
6. Kagan, A., Gordon, T., Rhoades, G. G., et al. Some factors related to coronary heart disease incidence in Honolulu Japanese men: The Honolulu Heart Study. *Int. J. Epidemiol. 4*:271, 1975.
7. Garrison, R. J., Wilson, P. W., Castelli, W. P., et al. Obesity and lipoprotein cholesterol in the Framingham offspring study. *Metabolism 29*:1055, 1980.
8. Kannell, E. B., Castelli, W. P., and Gordon, T. Cholesterol in the prediction of arteriosclerotic disease. *Ann. Intern. Med. 90*:85, 1979.
9. DeFronzo, R., Ferrannini, E., and Koivisto, V. New concepts in the pathogenesia and treatment of diabetes mellitus. Proceedings of a Symposium: The role of insulin resistance in the pathogenesis and treatment of noninsulin dependent diabetes mellitus. *Am. J. Med. 74*:52, 1983.

10. Kosaka, K., Hagura, E., and Kuzuya, T. Insulin response in equivocal and definite diabetes, with special reference to subjects who had mild glucose intolerance but later developed definite diabetes. *Diabetes* 26:944, 1977.
11. Himsworth, H. P, and Kerr, R. B. Insulin-sensitive and insulin-insensitive types of diabetes mellitus. *Clin. Sci.* 4:120, 1942.
12. Alford, R. P., Martin, F. L., and Pearson, M. J. The significance of interpretation of mildly abnormal oral glucose tolerance. *Diabetologia* 7:173, 1971.
13. Butterfield, W. J. H., and Whichelow, M. J. Peripheral glucose metabolism in control subjects and diabetic patients during glucose, glucose-insulin and insulin sensitivity tests. *Diabetologia* 1:43, 1965.
14. Jackson, R. A., Perry, G. Rogers, J., Advani, U., and Pikington, T. R. Relationship between the basal glucose concentration, glucose tolerance and forearm glucose uptake in maturity-onset diabetes. *Diabetes* 22:751, 1973.
15. Jackson, R. A., Peters, N., Advani, U., et al. Forearm glucose uptake during oral glucose tolerance test in normal subjects. *Diabetes* 22:442, 1973.
16. Zierler, K. L., and Pabinowitz, D. Roles of insulin and growth hormone, based on studies of forearm metabolism in man. *Medicine* 42:385, 1963.
17. Reaven, G. M., Bernstein, R., Davis, B., and Olefsky, J. M. Nonketotic diabetes mellitus; insulin deficiency or insulin resistance? *Am. J. Med.* 60:80, 1976.
18. Permutt, A., Chirgwin, J., Giddings, S., Kakita, K., and Rotwein, P. Insulin biosynthesis and diabetes mellitus. *Clin. Biochem.* 14:230, 1981.
19. DeFronzo, R. A., Soman, V., Sherwin, R. S., Hendler, R., and Felig, P. Insulin binding to monocytes and insulin action in human obesity, starvation, and refeeding. *J. Clin. Invest.* 62:204, 1978.
20. Kolterman, O. G., Insel, J., Saekow, M., and Olefsky, J. M Mechanism of insulin resistance in human obesity. *J. Clin. Invest.* 65:1272, 1980.
21. Holloszy, J. O., and Narahara, H. T. Enhanced permeability to sugar associated with muscle contraction, studies on the role of Ca^{++}. *J. Gen. Physiol.* 50:551, 1967.
22. Richter, E., Garetto, L. P., Goodman M. N., and Ruderman B. Muscle glucose metabolism following exercise in the rat: increased snesitivity to insulin. *J. Clin. Invest.* 69:785, 1982.

23. Zierler, K. L., and Rabinowitz, D. Roles of insulin and growth hormone, based on studies of forearm metabolism in man. *Medicine 42*: 285, 1963.

24. DeFronzo, R. A., Simonson, D., and Ferrannini, E. Hepatic and peripheral insulin resistance: a common feature in non-insulin dependent and insulin dependent diabetes. *Diabetologia 23*:313, 1982.

25. Olefsky, J. M., and Reaven, G. M. Insulin binding in diabetes. Relationship with plasma insulin levels and insulin sensitivity. *Diabetes 26*:680, 1977.

26. Kolterman, O. G., Gray, R. S., Griffin, J., et al. Receptor and postreceptor defects contribute to the insulin resistance in non-insulin dependent diabetes mellitus. *J. Clin. Invest. 68*:957, 1981.

27. Scarlett, J. A., Gray, R. S., Griffin, J., Olefsky, J. M., and Kilterman, O. G. Insulin treatment reverses insulin resistance of type II diabetes mellitus. *Diabetes Care 5*:353, 1982.

28. Savage, P. J., Bennion, L. J., Flock, E. V., et al. Diet induced improvement of abnormalities in insulin and glucagon secretion and in insulin receptor binding in diabetes mellitus. *J. Clin. Endocrinal. and Metab. 48*:999, 1979.

29. Genuth, S. M., Vertes, V., and Hazelton, I. Supplemental fasting in the treatment of obesity. In G. Bray (ed.), *Recent Advances in Obesity Research*. II. John Libbey and Co. Ltd., London, pp. 370–378, 1978.

30. Brunzell, J. D., Lerner, R. L., Porte, D. Jr., and Bierman, E. L. Effect of a fat free, high carbohydrate diet on diabetic subjects with fasting hyperglycemia. *Diabetes 23*:138, 1974.

31. Wall, J. R., Payke, D. A., and Oakly, W. F. Effect of carbohydrate restriction in obese diabetics: relationship of control to weight loss. *Br. Med. J. 1*:577, 1973.

32. Crapo, P. F., Kolterman, O. G., and Olefsky, J. M. Effects of oral fructose in normal, diabetic and impaired glucose tolerance subjects. *Diabetes Care 3*:575, 1980.

33. Crapo, P. A., Reaven, G., and Olefsky, J. M. Plasma glucose and insulin responses to orally administered simple and complex carbohydrates. *Diabetes 25*:741, 1976.

34. Akgum, S., and Ertel, N. H. A comparison of carbohydrate metabolism after sucrose, sorbitol and fructose meals in normal and diabetic subjects. *Diabetes Care 3*:582, 1980.

35. Jenkins, D. J. A., Leeds, A. R., Gassull, M. A., Cochet, B., and Alberti, K. G. M. M. Decrease in postprandial insulin and glucose concentrations by sugar and pectin. *Ann. Intern. Med. 86*:20, 1977.

36. Kiehm, T. G., Anderson, J. W., and Ward, K. Beneficial effects of high carbohydrate, high fiber diet on hyperglycemic diabetic men. *Am. J. Clin. Nutr. 29*:895, 1976.
37. Savage, P. J., Bennion, L. J., Flock, E. V., et al. Diet-induced improvement of abnormalities in insulin and glucagon secretion and in insulin receptor binding in diabetes mellitus. *J. Clin. Endocrinol. Metab. 48*: 999, 1979.
38. Naugulesparan, M., Savage, P. J., Bennion, L. J., Unger, R. H., and Bennett, P. H. Diminished effect of caloric restriction on control of hyperglycemia with increasing duration of type II mellitus. *J. Clin. Endocrinol. Metab. 53*:560, 1981.
39. Hadden, D. R., Montgomery, D. A., Skelly, R. J., et al. Maturity onset diabetes mellitus. *Br. Med. J. 3*:276, 1975.
40. Stanik, S., and Marcus, R. Insulin secretion improves following dietary control of plasma glucose in severely hyperglycemic obese patients. *Metabolism 29*:346, 1980.
41. Bec-Neilson, H., Pedersen, O., and Sorensen, N. S. Effects of dietary changes on cellular insulin binding and in vivo insulin sensitivity. *Metabolism 29*:482, 1980.
42. Newburgh, L. H. Control of hyperglycemia of obese diabetics by weight reduction. *Ann. Intern. Med. 17*:935, 1942.
43. Rudnick, P. A., and Taylor, K. W. Effect of prolonged carbohydrate restriction on serum insulin levels in mild diabetics. *Br. Med. J. 1*: 222, 1965.
44. Doar, J. W., Thompson, M. E., Wilde, C. E., and Sewell, C. E. Influence of treatment with diet alone on oral glucose tolerance test and plasma sugar and insulin levels in patients with maturity-onset diabetes mellitus. *Lancet 1*:1263, 1975.
45. Felber, J. P., Meyer, H. U., Curchod, B., Maeder, E., Pahud, P., and Jequier, E. Effect of a 3-day fast on glucose storage and oxidation in obese hyperinsulinemic diabetics. *Metabolism 30*:184, 1981.
46. Savage, P. J., Bennion, L., and Bennett, P. H. Normalization of insulin and glucagon secretion in Keton's-resistant diabetes mellitus with prolonged diet therapy. *J. C. E. and M. 49*:831, 1979.
47. Vranic, M., and Berger, M. Exercise and diabetes mellitus. *Diabetes 28*(supplement):147, 1979.
48. Pruett, E. D. R. Plasma insulin concentrations during prolonged work at near maximal oxygen uptake. *J. Appl. Physiol. 29*:155, 1970.
49. Felig, P., Wahren, J., Hendler, R., et al. Plasma glucagon levels in exercising man. *N. Engl. J. Med. 287*:184, 1972.

50. Galbo, H., Holst, J., and Christensen, N. J. Glucagon and plasma catecholamine responses to graded and prolonged exercise in man. *J. Appl. Physiol. 38*:70, 1975.

51. Christensen, N. J., Galbo, H., Hansen, J. F., Hess, B., Richter, E. A., and Trap-Jensen, J. Catecholamines and exercise. *Diabetes 28*(supplement):58, 1979.

52. Holloszy, J. O., and Narahara, H. T. Enhanced permeability to sugar associated with muscle contraction. Studies on the role of Ca^{++}. *J. Gen. Physiol. 50*:551, 1967.

53. Richter, E. A., Garetto, L. P., Goodman, M. N., and Ruderman, B. Muscle glucose metabolism following exercise in the rat: increased sensitivity to insulin. *J. Clin. Invest. 69*:785, 1982.

54. Wahren, J., Felig, P., and Hagenfeldt, L. Physical and fuel homeostasis in diabetes mellitus. *Diabetologia 14*:213, 1978.

55. Vranic, M., and Wrenshall, G. A. Exercise, insulin and glucose turnover in dogs. *Endocrinology 85*:165, 1969.

56. DeFronzo, R. A., Ferrannini, E., Sato, Y., Felig, P., and Wahren, J. Synergistic interaction between exercise and insulin on peripheral glucose metabolism. *J. Clin. Invest. 68*:1468, 1981.

57. Lohmann, D., Liebold, F., Heilmann, W., Senger, H., and Pohl, A. Diminished insulin response in highly trained athletes. *Metabolism 27*:521, 1978.

58. LeBlanc, J., Nadeau, A., and Boulay, M. Rousseau-Migneron, W. Effects of physical training and adiposity on glucose metabolism and 124I-insulin binding. *J. Appl. Physiol. 46*:235, 1979.

59. Bjorntorp, P., DeJounge, K., Sjostrom, L., and Sullivan, L. The effect of physical training on insulin production in obesity. *Metabolism 19*: 631, 1970.

60. Bjorntorp, P., Holm, G., Jacobsson, B., et al. Physical training in human hyperplastic obesity. IV. Effects on the hormonal status. *Metabolism 6*:319, 1977.

61. Soman, V. R., Koivisto, V. A., Delbert, D., Felig, P., and DeFonzo, R. A. Increased insulin sensitivity and insulin binding to monocytes after physical training. *N. Engl. J. Med. 301*:1200, 1979.

62. Olefsky, J. M., and Reaven, G. M. Effects of sulfonylurea therapy on insulin binding to mononuclear leukocytes of diabetic patients. *Am. J. Med. 60*:89, 1976.

63. Friedman, C. I., Falko, J. M., Patel, S., Kim, M. H., and Newman, H. A. I. Serum lipoprotein responses during active and stable weight reduction in reproductive obese females. *Clin. Res. 28*:152, 1980.

64. Schrott, H. G., Mason, E. E., and Printen, K. J. High density lipoprotein cholesterol changes in massive weight loss. *Clin. Res. 27*:227A, 1979.
65. Thompson, P. D., Jeffery, R. W., Wing, R. R., and Wood, P. D. Unexpected decrease in plasma high density lipoprotein cholesterol with weight loss. *American Journal of Clinical Nutrition 32*:2016, 1979.
66. Brownell, K. D., and Stunkard, A. J. Differential changes in plasma high-density lipoprotein-cholesterol levels in obese men and women during weight reduction. *Arch. Intern. Med. 141*:1142, 1981.
67. Streja, D. A., Boydo, E., and Rabkin, S. W. Changes in plasma high-density lipoprotein cholesterol concentration after weight reduction in grossly obese subjects. *British Medical Journal 281*:770, 1980.
68. Lopes-Virella, M. E. L., Stone, P. G., and Colwell, J. A. Serum high density lipoprotein in diabetic patients. *Diabetologia 13*:285, 1977.
69. Hartung, G. H., Foreyt, J. P., Mitchell, R. E., Mitchell, J. G., Reeves, R. S., and Gotto, A. M. Effect of alcohol intake on high-density lipoprotein cholesterol levels in runners and inactive men. *J.A.M.A. 249*: 747, 1983.
70. Hunt, J. C., Cooper, T., Frohlich, E. D., Gifford, R. W., Kaplan, N. M., Laragh, J. H., Maxwell, M. H., and Strong, C. G. *Dialogues in Hypertension.* Health Learning Systems, Inc., Bloomfield, N.J. p. 1, 1980.
71. Altschul, A. M., and Grommet, J. K. Food choices for lowering sodium intake. *Hypertension 4*(supplement III):111-116, 1982.
72. MacGregor, G. A., Best, F. E., Cam, J. M., Markandu, N. D., Elder, D. M., Sagnella, G. A., and Squires, M. Double-blind randomised crossover trial of moderate sodium restriction in essential hypertension. *Lancet 8*:268, 1982.
73. Dahl, L. K., Heine, M., and Thompson, K. Genetic influence of the kidneys in blood pressure, evidence from clironic reual homograples in rats with opposite predispositions to hypertension. *Arch. Res. 40*: 94, 1974.
74. Dietz, R., Schomig, A., Wolfgang, R., Strasser, R., BorwinLuth, J., Ganten, U., and Wolfgang, K. Contribution of the sympathetic nervous system to the hypertensive effect of a high sodium diet in stroke-prone spontaneously hypertensive rats. *Hypertension 4*:773, 1982.
75. Langford, H. Drug and dietary intervention in hypertension. *Hypertension 4*(supplement III):166, 1982.
76. Reisin, E., Abel, R., and Modan, M. Effect of weight loss without salt restriction on the reduction of blood pressure in overweight hypertensive subjects. *New Engl. J. Med. 298*:1, 1978.

77. Sowers, J. R., Nyby, M., Stern, N., Beck, F., Baron, S., Catania, R., and Vlachis, N. Blood pressure and hormone changes associated with weight reduction in the obese. *Hypertension 4*:686, 1982.

78. Sowers, J. R., Whitfield, L. A., Catania, R. A., Tuck, M. L., Dornfeld, L., Stern, N., and Maxwell, M. Role of the sympathetic nervous system in blood pressure maintenance in obesity. *Journal of Clinical Endocrinology and Metabolism 54*:1181, 1982.

79. Danforth, E. Jr., Horton, F. S., O'Connell, N., Sims, E. A. H., Gurger, A. G., Ingbar, S. H., Braverman, L., and Vageuakis, A. G. Dietary-induced alteration in thyroid hormone metabolism during over nutrition. *J. Clin. Invest. 64*:1336, 1979.

80. Besareb, A., Silva, P., Laudsberg, L., and Epstein, F. H. Effect of catecholamines on tubular function in the isolated perfused rat kidney. *Am. J. Physiol. 233*:F29, 1977.

81. Young, J. B., Rowe, J. W., Palotta, J. A., Sparrow, D., and Laudsberg, L. Enhanced plasma norepinephrine response to upright posture and oral glucose administration in elderly human subjects. *Metabolism 29*: 532, 1980.

82. Rowe, J. W., Young, J. B., Minaker, K. L., Stevens, A. L., Pallottia, J., and Landsberg, L. Effect of insulin and glucose infusions on sympathetic nervous system activity in normal man. *Diabetes 30*:219, 1981.

83. Andre, R., and Crabge, J. Stimulation by insulin of active sodium transport by toad skin; influence of celdesterene and vasopressin. *Arch. Int. Physiol. Biochem. 74*:538, 1966.

84. DeFronzo, R. A., Cooke, C. R., Andres, R., Faloona, G., and Davis, P. J. The effect of insulin on reval handling of sodium, potassium calcium and phosphate in man. *J. Clin. Invest. 55*:845, 1975.

85. Cahill, C. F. Starvation in man. *New Engl. J. Med. 282*:660, 1970.

86. Tuck, M. L., Sowers, J., Dornfeld, L., Kledzik, G., and Maxwell, M. The effect of weight reduction on blood pressure, plasma renin activity, and plasma aldosterone levels in obese patients. *New Engl. J. Med. 304*:930, 1981.

87. DeFronzo, R. A., Goldberg, M., and Agus, Z. The effects of glucose and insulin reval electrolyte transport. *J. Clin. Invest. 58*:85, 1976.

88. Bjorntorp, P., DeJounga, K., Sjostrom, L., and Sullivan, L. The effect of physical training on insulin prodirection in obesity. *Metabolism 19*: 631, 1970.

89. Euler, U. S., and Hellner, S. Excretion of rioradrenaline and adrenaline in muscular work. *Acta Physiol. Scand. 26*:183, 1952.

90. Krotkiewski, M., Mandroukas, M., Sjostrom, L. M., Sullivan, H., and Bjorntorp, P. Effects of long-term physical training on body fat, metabolism and blood pressure in obesity. *Metabolism 28*:649, 1979.

91. Hovel, M. F. The experimental evidence for weight-loss treatment of essential hypertension: a critical review. *Am. J. Publ. Health 72*:359, 1982.

92. Puska, P., Nissinen, A., Vartiainen, E., Dougherty, R., Mutanen, M., Iacono, J., Korhonen, H., Pietinen, P., Leino, U., Moisio, S., and Huttunen, J. Controlled randomised trial of the effect of dietary fat on blood pressure. *Lancet 8314*:5, 1983.

4

Clinical Assessment of the Obese Individual

Cecilia Pemberton

INTRODUCTION

The word "obesity" is derived from the Latin *ob*, meaning over, and *edere*, meaning to eat. The longstanding bias that obesity is simply the result of overeating is reflected in the derivation of the word. In fact, the idea that obesity is the result of ingestion of more calories than expended has become a socially accepted, and often medically reinforced truism. However, the energy equation should be viewed as simply a statement of the *conditions* required for deposition of lipids in adipocytes and not the *cause* of the caloric imbalance. Focus on energy balance, without consideration of the underlying causes, is a deterrant to selection of potentially effective treatment

Copyright © 1984 by Spectrum Publications, Inc., *Evaluation and Treatment of Obesity*, edited by J. Storlie and H. A. Jordan.

options and perpetuates an often inappropriate attitude of blame toward the obese individual.

The factors causing or contributing to obesity are numerous, but not yet clearly elucidated. However, there is sufficient information to indicate that the obese are a diverse group with many differences [1]. A pitfall in treatment of obesity is the tendency toward bias of recommendations according to the background or strengths of the clinician or counselor. The inclination is to offer services in which one is trained, regardless of the needs of the individual patient. Those from the rigid medical mold are likely to advise simple caloric restriction. Conversely, behavior modification is often recommended by its proponents with little attention to diet. A comprehensive assessment of the multiple factors contributing to the development of obesity can take one out of the setting of simply making exhortations to eat less, exercise more, or develop better eating habits, and can allow an approach to treatment of obesity in a more rational, objective manner with less implication of human frailty and lack of will-power. The purpose of multifactorial assessment is primarily to influence intervention through choice of, or emphasis, on treatment modality and goal of treatment. Second, collection of clinical data can contribute to improved understanding of the etiology of obesity.

ANTHROPOMETRIC AND BODY MEASUREMENTS

Measurement of height and weight are essential baseline data, but may be a poor indication of obesity [2,3,4]. Conscientious attention to technique can make skinfold thickness measurements a reliable indicator of percentage of body fat, at least in races studied and in those not grossly obese [2,5,6]. However, among other limitations, skinfold measurements are not a good indicator of slow, gradual weight loss [7,8]. Skinfold measurements and estimation of percentage of body fat may be appropriately used to identify the goal of weight loss and exercise to reduce body fat to a lower level for cardiovascular benefit.

Anthropometric measurements and somatotyping may be useful in assessing the degree of obesity and identifying other characteristics, such as type of fat distribution, whether central or peripheral, which can infer expected morbidity and prognosis [9,10]. Central obesity tends to be associated with more metabolic abnormalities; peripheral obesity tends to result from hyperplasia.

ASSOCIATED DISEASES

Because of the high prevalence of diabetes, hypertension, and hyperlipidemia in obese persons, clinical and biochemical evaluation of these diseases should be included as part of an overall assessment [11,12,13,14].

The number of obese individuals who have recognized genetically transmitted obesity syndromes, such as the Laurence–Moon–Bardet–Biedl and the Prader–Willi syndromes, is thought to be relatively small [15], but the possibility should not be ignored. Other endocrine system dysfunction, such as Cushing's disease and thyroid disorders, may cause obesity. As a working guide, individuals who are morbidly obese, without a family history of obesity, should have thorough medical evaluation for obesity secondary to other diseases. The frequency of obesity within families is high. More than sixty percent of obese individuals have at least one parent who is obese [16]; the frequency is probably much greater when grandparents and siblings are included.

METABOLIC RATE

Measurement of basal metabolic rate is useful for discussion of calorie expenditure and projecting rate of weight loss with calorie restriction. In individuals who have a relatively low resting metabolic rate (i.e., ten to fifteen percent less than predicted or less than 1200 to 1300 kilocalories), calorie restriction alone will be only marginally effective and advice to improve

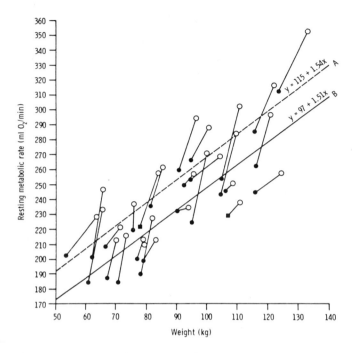

Figure 1. Resting metabolic rate and body weight in 27 obese women before (open circles) and after (closed circles) 3 weeks on a diet supplying 800 kcal daily [20].

eating behaviors will be inadequate. In these individuals, one goal of treatment can be increased calorie expenditure through increased physical activity or possibly through changes away from abberant eating patterns.

The metabolic rate is not a constant and the variance within an individual is rarely known. It is known that the resting metabolic rate decreases in starvation [17] and with caloric restriction in dieting [18]. A ten to forty-five percent decrease in basal metabolic rate has been reported, depending upon the severity and duration of the caloric restriction [18] (Figure 1). Bray [19] has shown that metabolic rate can decrease by as much as twenty percent in as little as two weeks with reduction of calorie intake from 3500 kilocalories to 450 kilocalories per

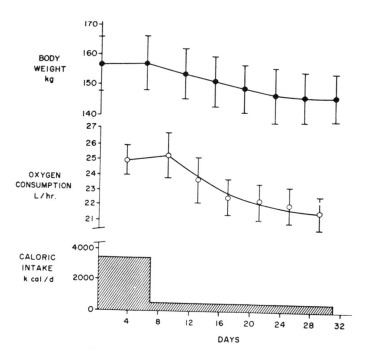

Figure 2. Effect of caloric restriction on oxygen consumption of 6 obese patients. After 1 week on a diet of 3500 kcal/day caloric intake reduced to 450 kcal/day. Body weight declined but the drop in oxygen uptake was proportionally faster, representing a fall of 15 percent by the end of 2 weeks [19].

day, and that the decline begins within 24 to 48 hours after the calorie restriction begins, but returns to previous levels with increased calorie intake. The decrease in metabolic rate with calorie restriction cannot be attributed to decrease in body weight since the decline in metabolic rate is proportionally faster (Figure 2). Garrow [20] has reported that, with successive episodes of caloric restriction, metabolic rate falls more rapidly with each episode and that return to baseline levels takes longer each time the restriction ends. Efforts to reduce weight through severe caloric restriction may prove to be

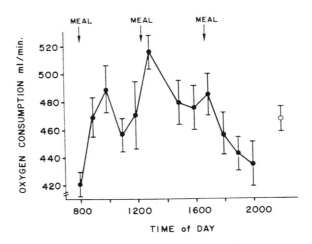

Figure 3. Oxygen consumption in one obese patient throughout the day. The rise in oxygen consumption after each of the meals is evident. This rise was smallest after the evening meal. The open circle on the right is the mean figure for resting metabolism of this patient [24].

counterproductive because of the potential for adaptive changes in energy expenditure through decreased metabolic rate. Repeated attempts at stringent dieting may compound the problem through a progressively slower return of metabolic rate to normal levels.

It can be postulated that the composition of a low calorie diet, particularly if the diet is very low in or almost devoid of carbohydrate, can also lower the metabolic rate through changes in thyroid hormone levels. A decrease in triiodothyronine (T_3) and an increase in the inactive form, reverse triiodothyronine (rT_3), have been documented in starvation [17], in weight loss with dieting [21], and with carbohydrate restriction [22], especially when the calorie intake is at or below maintenance levels [23]. It is unclear whether the decrease in T_3 is the cause of decreased metabolic rate, but it undoubtedly contributes. Refeeding with carbohydrate after fasting, reverses the levels of T_3 and rT_3 to euthyroid levels. The effect of varying levels of carbohydrate on thyroid hormone levels and basal metabolic rate have not been thoroughly investigated, but it can be speculated from existing data that disproportionate restriction of carbohydrate in low calorie diets may accentuate the propensity toward lowered metabolic rate. The decrease in metabolic rate with caloric restriction and with minimal carbohydrate intake may help explain the rigid dietary restrictions that some individuals find necessary for weight maintenance after weight loss on very low calorie, low carbohydrate diets.

Diurnal variations in metabolic rate are known [20,24], but the factors influencing them are not well documented. A progressive decline in metabolic rate has been documented from day to day with severe caloric restriction, and it is likely that there are changes in metabolic rate over shorter periods of time. One or two hours after a meal there is an increase in metabolic rate which is about forty percent above basal at its peak and averages ten percent above baseline over a period of about six hours [20]. There is limited evidence that the rise in metabolic rate is less after the evening meal [24]. It can be speculated that the night eating pattern, in which the majority of calories are consumed over a relatively short period of time in the evening hours, results in an overall decrease in metabolic rate. The mechanism may be through decreased basal metabolic rate or lessened postprandial increases in metabolic rate because of lessened frequency of food ingestion (Figure 3).

Basal or resting rate are the indices measured most frequently in the clinical setting. The data are preliminary, but theoretically measurement of postprandial metabolic rate could serve as an indicator of defects in dietary thermogenesis, the calorie expenditure induced by ingestion and metabolism of food. There is some indication of a lessened thermogenic response to food intake in obesity [20,25,26,27,28].

FAMILY HISTORY

Review of the prevalence of obesity in the individual's family is necessary for recommendation of a goal weight which is achievable and compatible with optimum health.

There is a close association within families for height, and a positive but less strong correlation for weight and fatness [16,29]. The degree to which heredity and environmental factors contribute to this resemblance is disputed. Twin studies and family studies indicate that there is a heritable component but the evidence is far from unequivocal [29]. Recent studies of HLA antigens in families with a high prevalence of obesity have given further support to the possible existence of a genetic form of obesity [30]. Adoption study designs have been less than ideal. Some have reported that environment is the most important influence, while other adoption studies have indicated that heritability is more important [29].

Family history is important regardless of the manner through which it affects weight. The goal weight for obese individuals with a strong positive family history of obesity should be made in the context of genetic inheritance and environmental background of the individual and less in reference to standard height–weight tables. For individuals with a strong positive family history of obesity, an achievable and realistic goal weight may be substantially greater than reference standards.

DEVELOPMENTAL HISTORY

Review of the age of onset of obesity and changes in weight throughout adult years is necessary to recommend a goal weight which is compatible with optimum health, but not necessarily statistical standards.

The developmental history provides suggestive evidence regarding hypercellular or hypertrophic obesity. An actual diagnosis of hypercellular obesity can only be made using techniques that are not readily available for measurement of total body fat and size or weight of the adipocyte. However, a presumptive diagnosis of hypercellular obesity can be made on a clinical basis when the age of onset of obesity is in childhood or adolescence [31,32,33]. The prognosis of weight loss in hypercellular obesity is poor, or perhaps it is that the expectations are

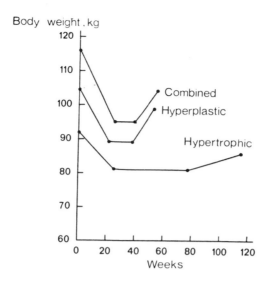

Figure 4. Schematic summary of the mean results of treatment of patients with combined (hypertrophic and hyperplastic), hyperplastic, and hypertrophic obesity [34].

too great. Individuals with hypercellular obesity, as compared to those with hypertrophic obesity, lose weight more rapidly and often achieve a greater weight loss but also have a greater degree of relapse and subsequent weight gain (Figure 4) [34].

This phenomenon has been interpreted that a decrease in lipid content of the adipocyte beyond an unknown level is physiologically abnormal and meets with physiologic resistance. Therefore, only modest weight reduction, or even the prevention of further weight increases, should be attempted when a presumptive diagnosis of hypercellular obesity is made. The focus should be on attainment of physiologically realistic conditions.

The critical time theory proposed that development of hypercellular obesity took place only at critical stages of development in childhood and adolescence, and that weight gain in adults was due only to hypertrophy of fat cells without formation of new fat cells. Recognition of hypercellularity in

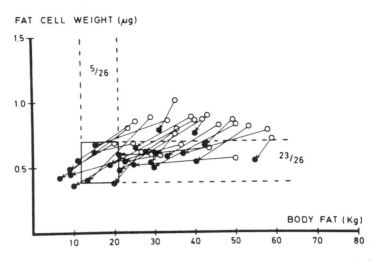

Figure 5. Body fat and average fat cell weight of obese women before treatment (open symbols). Changes after failure to reduce further in body weight on an energy reduced diet (arrows and closed symbols). The rectangle denotes the mean ± SD of values of controls [31].

adult onset obesity has since brought about revision of the critical time theory. Current theory holds that attainment of a maximum cell size could trigger proliferation of new adipose cells, under certain conditions, and at any age. The previously described periods in childhood and adolescence may be those stages of development where hyperplasia of adipocytes is more likely to occur [33].

Weight reduction appears to cease when fat cell size reaches normal values, regardless of fat cell number. A decrease in fat cell number has not been demonstrated in short term weight reduction of approximately one year; it is unknown whether long term sustained weight reduction would decrease the number of adipocytes. Sjöström [31] (Figure 5) has referred to this phenomenon as a biologic trap—each time the body weight increases over previous levels, there is the potential for development of new fat cells, which do not decrease in number in short periods of weight reduction. Theoretically, each period of weight gain could set the subsequent physiologically attainable weight at a higher level. This theory may help explain the weight gain that occurs in adults in almost staircase type fashion and is highly refractory. Obviously, efforts for these individuals to attempt to reduce weight to an arbitrary or previous low level, such as weight at age 20, is inappropriate. The circumstances associated with the development of hypercellular and hypertrophic obesity in adult onset obesity remain unclear, but the possibility of hypercellular obesity in adults should temper our expectations.

USUAL DIET AND MEAL PATTERN

Nutritional assessment should include: (1) an overview of the frequency of eating, particularly the meal–snack pattern; (2) the variety of foods eaten with attention to consumption of fat, sugar, and alcohol; and (3) a general estimate of quantity. The role of diet in the etiology of obesity remains unclear. Reports of eating habits and food choices of obese and non-obese groups have provided conflicting data but, in general, have not substantiated the view that obese people have major differences in food choice or eating patterns [35,36,37,38]. Nonetheless, an assessment of the obese individual's usual diet and eating pattern can give some indication of areas where there is potential for change.

The assumption that most people who have dieted have adequate knowledge of nutrition is erroneous. The abundance of bizarre fad diets has left many people with false and misleading notions. Individuals who have a distorted meal–snack pattern and either snack frequently or eat only one large meal per day generally need specific dietary guidelines to plan meals of appropriate composition and portion size. Individuals who have followed multiple very low calorie diets with subsequent periods of rebound overeating often have a distorted concept of their calorie needs and are more likely, on their own, to plan a diet that is overly restrictive. While per capita consumption of calories has decreased, the proportion of fat has increased since the early 1900s [39]. Since fat is such an insidious part of our

food suply, individuals who have tended toward a high fat intake, either through excessive use of added fats, fat in cooking,
or inherently high fat foods, need specific dietary guidelines
to reverse the composition toward a higher carbohydrate, lower
fat diet. Individuals who have tended to be conscientious in
their choice of foods and eating habits can benefit from guidelines relating their calorie intake and energy expenditure and
then choosing small cumulative changes. Although diet alone
has proven to be unsuccessful in weight management [40,41,
42], diet—food choice, quantity, preparation, and meal pattern—
should not be excluded from weight management efforts. The
amount of dietary advice that the obese individual requires will
depend on the individual's knowledge base, whether accurate or
erroneous, and the degree of change required.

PHYSICAL ACTIVITY PATTERN

An assessment of the physical activity pattern should include both routine and scheduled or recreational activity.
There is conflicting evidence, but the overall suggestion
from many studies is that obese children are as active as their
nonobese peers. However, obese adults are likely to be less
active than nonobese adults [43]. The implication is that inactivity is more likely a consequence than an initial cause of
obesity. The primary role of inactivity may be in the per-
petuation of excess weight and further weight gain.
Almost all obese individuals can benefit from increased
physical activity [43,44]. However, the rationale for increasing
physical activity and the anticipated effect will vary. Physical
activity has the obvious effect of increased calorie expenditure
through movement of the body. The metabolic rate is increased
during the performance of physical activity and for a period of
time afterwards. There is speculation that physical activity may
counteract some of the decrease in metabolic rate which
accompanies caloric restriction [43]. Moderate physical activity
is thought to act as an appetite suppressant since increase in
activity from sedentary to moderate is accompanied by a

decrease in calorie intake [43,45]. Physical activity may also be useful as an alternative to overeating in response to stress.

RESPONSE TO EXTERNAL CUES

It has been suggested that the obese are more responsive than the nonobese to external or environmental cues to eating and that obese individuals eat primarily in response to these cues rather than to internal physiologic stimuli or hunger [46]. This hypothesis set the background for behavior modification efforts to teach stimulus control in an effort to minimize the number of external cues that would elicit eating behavior. There is evidence to support the externality theory, but there is also evidence that most people are responsive to some external cues and that some people in all weight categories are more responsive and others less so [47,48]. The difference in responsiveness to external cues between the obese and nonobese may not be as great as once thought [49].

Based on clinical judgement of responsiveness to external cues, the recommendations for treatment will vary so that those who are highly responsive to external cues are taught stimulus control through behavior modification, and so that those who exhibit less overt responsiveness to external cues emphasize other aspects of weight control.

RESTRAINED EATING

Restrained eating is the voluntary and intentional restriction of food [50,51,52]. Restraint is measured by the amount of conscious thought devoted to weight and food and how frequently one is dieting. People in all weight categories vary in the degree of restrained eating behavior; obesity does not correlate with restraint. Restrained eating has been associated with overeating prior to a period of anticipated food deprivation [53] or following circumstances which induce the person to eat more than usual or planned (Figure 6). The cause of this

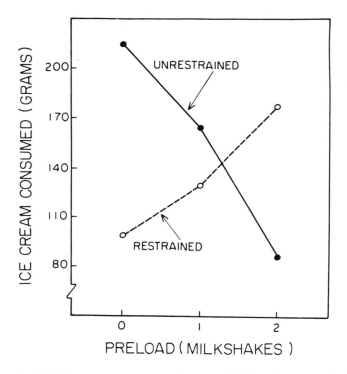

Figure 6. Ad libitum consumption (ice cream) following controlled and varied quantity of preload (milk shakes) in restrained and unrestrained eaters [50].

phenomenon is open to speculation. A possible interpretation is that the prospect that food restriction elicits overeating; "going off the diet" causes the restrained eater to lose his or her resolve. The restrained eating phenomenon may help explain the cycle of dieting and binging and the rebound overeating following severe caloric restriction.

Awareness of the restrained eating phenomenon is useful to help alleviate concerns of individuals with this behavior. Specific dietary guidelines, presenting only a modest calorie deficit, may be helpful in establishing a less disparate eating cycle.

PERSONALITY

Efforts to identify personality characteristics unique to obesity have, in general, been unsuccessful [54,55,56,57]. Currently, efforts are directed toward identifying differences between various subgroups. There is some indication that those who are morbidly obese exhibit more traits of addictive behavior [58] and tend to deal with frustration internally, where as those who are moderately obese tend to deal with frustration more aggressively and externally [59]. These data should be viewed as preliminary, and care should be taken that they are interpreted with caution at this time.

Differences in internal–external locus of control have not been identified in development of obesity in childhood [60], but there is evidence that a predominantly internal locus of control is positively correlated with success in various weight reduction programs [61,62,63]. It can be speculated that assessment of internal–external locus of control could be used as a predictor of success and, potentially, to direct individuals to types of programs for which they have the best promise of success.

An individual is described as having inner directed or internal control if an event is perceived as contingent upon that individual's behavior. In contrast, an individual's perception of an event as not being entirely contingent upon the individual's action, is described as externally controlled, or in common terms, the result of luck, chance, or fate. Those individuals with a greater degree of internal control are more likely to succeed in programs which emphasize self direction and self reinforcement; those individuals with a greater component of external control may require more guidance, reinforcement, and support from the clinician or counselor. Consideration of the individual's internal–external locus of control may help one better direct obese individuals to appropriate treatment styles. (For a more in depth discussion of these issues, refer to Storlie, Chapter 6).

PSYCHIATRIC DISTURBANCES

The presence and nature of psychiatric disturbances in obese persons should be considered on an individual basis. Depression and anxiety may be somewhat less common when comparing broad groupings of obese and nonobese segments of the population. However, within the diverse group of the obese, there are segments, particularly young women, for whom anxiety and depression may be more prevelant [65]. Obesity and psychiatric disturbances are not necessarily causally related. A causal relationship is not unidirectional; obesity may be an outcome of psychiatric disturbances, and obesity itself may heighten anxiety and depression in some individuals [66].

Dieting can precipitate depression in some individuals [67, 68]. There is accumulating evidence that restrained eaters, or dieters, are hyperemotional, overeating in response to emotional stimuli in the environment, as compared to unrestrained eaters [50]. These responses to dieting are difficult to interpret, but it may be that dieting, for some individuals, is a stressor, a source of frustration and a drain on the ability to cope with emotional stresses [50].

For obese individuals who have psychiatric disturbances, or who have had periods of depression or unusual anxiety with previous dieting efforts, it seems prudent to temper treatment recommendations so that the demands of the diet or behavior changes are modest and achievable without undue stress. Periodic followup for reassurance, support and possible revision of diet and behavior recommendations may be particularly important for this type of patient.

COMPLICATING CONDITIONS—MEDICATIONS

There are reports in the literature of a wide variety of drugs causing changes in food consumption and body weight when administered for quite different purposes. Among these are minor tranquilizers, antidepressants, and antipsychotic drugs [69]. Among the minor tranquilizers, the benzodiazepines, diazepam (Valium) and chlordiazepoxide (Librium) have been found to cause a dramatic increase in food intake in a variety of animal species. Patients on the antidepressant amitriptyline (Elavil) have displayed carbohydrate craving and weight gain which subsides with discontinuation of the medication. Weight gain has also been associated with the antipsychotic drug lithium.

Consideration should be given to the prescription of medications which have the additional effect of increased food intake or weight gain, so that treatment of one disorder does not exacerbate another. When such medications are indicated, the treatment goal of obesity may need to be tempered. It may be possible to achieve only a very slow weight loss. In some instances, the goal may be to prevent further weight gain.

SUMMARY

Aspects of clinical assessment of the obese individual have been discussed with reference to effect on choice of optimum treatment modality, and on establishing a goal weight that is physiologically attainable and compatible with optimum health.

REFERENCES

1. Sims, E. A. Characterization of the syndromes of obesity. In *Diabetes Mellitus and Obesity.* Edited by B. N. Brodoff, S. J. Bleicher, Baltimore, Williams and Wilkins. 1982.
2. Bray, G. A. Who are the obese? In *The Obese Patient*, Vol. IX in the series Major Problems in Internal Medicine. Philadelphia, W. B. Saunders, Co. 1976.
3. Grande, F. Assessment of body fat in man. In *Obesity in Perspective.* Edited by G. A. Bray. Dept. of HEW Publication No. (NIH) 75-708. 1973.
4. Lee, J., Kolonel, L. N., and Hinds, M. W. The cause of an inappropriate weight-height derived index of obesity can produce misleading results. *Internat. J. Obesity* 6:233, 1982.

5. Durnin, J. V. G. A., and Womersley, J. Body fat assessed from skinfold thickness: measurements on 481 men and women aged from 16 to 72 years. *Br. J. Nutr. 32*:77, 1974.

6. Franzini, L. R., and Grimes, W. B. Skinfold measures as the criterion of change in weight control studies. *Behav. Therapy 7*:256, 1976.

7. Bray, G. A., et al. Use of anthropometric measures to assess weight loss. *Am. J. Clin. Nutr. 31*:769, 1978.

8. Johnson, W. G., and Stalonas, P. Measuring skinfold thickness—a cautionary note. *Addictive Behaviors 2*:105, 1977.

9. Vague, J. The degree of masculine differentiation of obesities: a factor determining predisposition to diabetes, atherosclerosis, gout and uric calculous disease. *Am. J. Clin. Nutr. 4*:20, 1956.

10. Aswell, M., Chinn, S., Stalley, S., and Garrow, J. S. Female fat distribution—a simple classification based on two circumference measurements. *Internat. J. Obesity 6*:143, 1982.

11. Bray, G. A., and Teague, R. J. An algorithm for medical evaluation of the obese patient. In *Obesity*. Edited by A. J. Stunkard. Philadelphia, W. B. Saunders, Co. 1980.

12. Bray, G. A. The risks and disadvantages of obesity. In *The Obese Patient*, Vol. IX in the series Major Problems in Internal Medicine. Philadelphia, W. B. Saunders, Co. 1976.

13. Van Itallie, T. B. Obesity; adverse effects. *Am. J. Clin. Nutr. 32*:2723, 1979.

14. Larsson, B., Björntorp, P., and Tibblin, G. The health consequences of moderate obesity. *Internat. J. Obesity 5*:97, 1981.

15. Bray, G. A. Experimental and clinical forms of obesity. In *The Obese Patient*, Vol. IX in the series Major Problems in Internal Medicine. Philadelphia, W. B. Saunders, Co. 1976.

16. Garn, S. M., et al. Effect of remaining family members on fatness prediction. *Am. J. Clin. Nutr. 34*:148, 1981.

17. Cahill, G. F., Jr. Starvation in man. In *Clinics in Endocrinology and Metabolism*, Vol. 5, No. 2, Obesity. Edited by M. J. Albrink. London, W. B. Saunders, Ltd. 1976.

18. Apfelbaum, M. Influence of level of energy intake on energy expenditure in man. In *Obesity in Perspective*. Edited by G. A. Bray. Dept. of HEW Publication No. (NIH) 75-708. 1973.

19. Bray, G. A. The effect of calorie restriction on energy expenditure in obese patients. *Lancet 2*:397, 1969.

20. Garrow, J. S. Factors affecting energy output. In *Energy Balance and Obesity in Man*, 2nd edition. Amsterdam, Elsevier/North-Holland Biomedical Press. 1978.

21. Bray, G. A., Fisher, D. A., and Chapra, I. J. Relation of thyroid hormones to body weight. *Lancet 1*:1206, 1976.
22. Danforth, E., et al. Dietary-induced alterations in thyroid hormone metabolism during overnutrition. *J. Clin. Invest. 64*:1336, 1979.
23. Davidson, M. B., and Chapra, I. J. Effects of carbohydrate and non-carbohydrate sources of calories in plasma 3, 5, 3'-triiodothyronine concentrations in man. *J. Clin. Endo. Metab. 48*:577, 1979.
24. Bray, G. A., et al. Relationship between oxygen consumption and body composition of obese patients. *Metabolism 19*:418, 1970.
25. Sims, E. A. Experimental obesity, dietary induced thermogenesis, and their clinical implications. In *Clinics in Endocrinology and Metabolism*, Vol. 5, No. 2, Obesity. Edited by M. J. Albrink. London, W. B. Saunders, Ltd. 1976.
26. Danforth, E., Jr. Dietary induced thermogenesis: control of energy expenditure. *Life Sciences 28*:1821, 1981.
27. Shetty, P. S., et al. Postprandial thermogenesis in obesity. *Clin. Sci. 60*:519, 1981.
28. Bray, G. A. Energy expenditure. In *The Obese Patient*, Vol. IX in the series Major Problems in Internal Medicine. Philadelphia, W. B. Saunders, Co. 1976.
29. Foch, T. T., and McClearn, G. E. Genetics, body weight and obesity. In *Obesity*. Edited by A. J. Stunkard. Philadelphia, W. B. Saunders, Co. 1980.
30. Apfelbaum, M., et al. Genetic approach of family obesity: study of HLA antigens in 10 families and 86 unrelated obese subjects. *Biomedic. 33*:98, 1980.
31. Sjöström, L. Fat cells and body weight. In *Obesity*. Edited by A. J. Stunkard. Philadelphia, W. B. Saunders, Co. 1980.
32. Hirsch, J., and Batchelor, B. Adipose tissue cellularity in human obesity. In *Clinics in Endocrinology and Metabolism*, Vol. 5, No. 2, Obesity. Edited by M. J. Albrink. London, W. B. Saunders, Ltd. 1976.
33. Björntorp, P. Development of adipose tissue. In *The Body Weight Regulatory System: Normal and Disturbed Mechanisms*. Edited by L. A. Cioffi, W. P. T. James, and T. B. Van Itallie. New York, Raven Press. 1981.
34. Krotkiewski, M., Sjöström, L., and Björntorp, P. Adipose tissue cellularity in relation to prognosis for weight reduction. *Internat. J. Obesity 1*:395, 1977.
35. Mahoney, M. J. The obese eating style: bites, beliefs and behavior modification. *Addictive Behaviors 1*:47, 1975.

36. Stunkard, A., and Kaplan, D. Eating in public places: a review of reports of direct observation of eating behavior. *Internat. J. Obesity* *1*:89, 1977.
37. Rosenthal, B. S., and Marx, R. D. Differences in eating patterns of successful and unsuccessful dieters, untreated overweight and normal weight individuals. *Addictive Behaviors 3*:129, 1978.
38. Edelman, B. Binge eating in normal weight and overweight individuals. *Psychol. Reports 49*:739, 1981.
39. Friend, B., Page, L., and Martson, R. Food consumption patterns in the United States: 1090-1976. In *Nutrition Lipids and Coronary Heart Disease*. Edited by R. Levy, et al. New York, Raven Press. 1979.
40. Bray, G. A. The myth of diet in management of obesity. *Am. J. Clin. Nutr. 23*:1141, 1970.
41. Glennon, J. A. Weight reduction—an enigma. *Arch. Intern. Med. 118*: 1, 1966.
42. Stunkard, A. J., and McLaren-Hume, M. The results of treatment of obesity. *Arch. Intern. Med. 103*:79, 1959.
43. Brownell, K. D., and Stunkard, A. J. Physical activity in the development and control of obesity. In *Obesity*. Edited by A. J. Stunkard. Philadelphia, W. B. Saunders, Co. 1980.
44. Björntorp, P. Exercise in the treatment of obesity. In *Clinics in Endocrinology and Metabolism*, Vol. 5, No. 2, Obesity. Edited by M. J. Albrink. London. W. B. Saunders, Ltd. 1976.
45. Woo, R., Garrow, J. S., and Pi-Sunyer, F. X. Effect of exercise on spontaneous calorie intake in obesity. *Am. J. Clin. Nutr. 36*:470, 1982.
46. Rodin, J., and Slochowier, J. Externality in the nonobese: effects of environment responsiveness on weight. *J. Person. Social Psychol. 33*:338, 1976.
47. Rodin, J. The externality theory today. In *Obesity*. Edited by A. J. Stunkard. Philadelphia, W. B. Saunders, Co. 1980.
48. Meyers, A. W., Stunkard, A. J., and Coll, M. Food accessibility and food choice. *Arch. Gen. Psychiat. 37*:1133, 1980.
49. Rodin, J. Current status of the internal–external hypothesis for obesity. *Am. Psychol. 36*:361, 1981.
50. Herman, C. P., and Polivy, J. Restrained eating . In *Obesity*. Edited by A. J. Stunkard. Philadelphia, W. B. Saunders, Co. 1980.

51. Stunkard, A. J. "Restrained eating": what it is and a new scale to measure it. In *The Body Weight Regulatory System: Normal and Disturbed Mechanisms.* Edited by L. A. Cioffi, W. P. T. James, and T. B. Van Itallie. New York, Raven Press. 1981.
52. Gormally, J., et al. The assessment of binge eating severity among obese persons. *Addictive Behaviors 7*:47, 1982.
53. Lowe, M. G. The role of anticipated deprivation in overeating. *Addictive Behaviors 7*:103, 1982.
54. Weinberg, N., Mendelson, M., and Stunkard, A. A failure to find distinctive personality features on a group of obese men. *Am. J. Psych. 117*:1035, 1961.
55. Stuart, R. B., and Davis, B. *Slim Chance in a Fat World.* Champaign, Ill., Research Press. 1972.
56. Johnson, S. F., Swenson, W. M., and Gastineau, C. F. Personality characteristics in obesity, relation of MMPI profile and age of onset of obesity to success in weight reduction. *Am. J. Clin. Nutr. 29*:626, 1976.
57. Höllstrom, T., and Napper, H. Obesity in women in relation to mental illness, social factors and personality traits. *J. Psychomatic Res. 25*: 75, 1981.
58. Leon, G. R., Kolotkin, R., and Korgeski, G. McCandrew addiction scale and other MMPI characteristics associated with obesity, anorexia and smoking behavior. *Addictive Behaviors 4*:401, 1979.
59. Igoin, L., and Apfelbaum, M. Differences in tolerance to frustration between moderately obese and severely obese subjects. *Internat. J. Obesity 6*:227, 1982.
60. Geller, S. E., Keane, T. M., and Scheirer, C. J. Delay of gratification, locus of control and eating patterns in obese and nonobese children. *Addictive Behaviors 6*:9, 1981.
61. Goldney, R. D., and Cameron, E. Locus of control as a predictor of attendance and success in the management of obesity. *Internat. J. Obesity 5*:39, 1981.
62. Kincey, J. Internal-external control and weight loss in the obese: predictive and discriminant validity and some possible clinical implications. *J. Clin. Psychol. 37*:100, 1981.
63. Chevez, E. I., and Michaels, A. C. Evaluation of health locus of control for obesity treatment. *Psychol. Reports 47*:709, 1980.
64. Rotter, J. B. Generalized expectancies for internal versus external control of reinforcement. *Psychol. Mongr. 80*:whole no. 609, 1966.

65. Crisp, A. H., et al. "Jolly fat" revisited. *J. Psychosomatic Res. 24*:233, 1980.
66. Bruch, H. *Eating Disorders: Obesity, Anorexia Nervosa and the Person Within.* New York, Basic Books, Inc. 1973.
67. Stunkard, A. J. The "dieting depression." *Am. J. Med. 23*:77, 1957.
68. Stunkard, A. J., and Rush, J. Dieting and depression re-examined. *Ann. Intern. Med. 81*:526, 1974.
69. Blundell, J. E. Pharmacological adjustments of the mechanisms underlying feeding and obesity. In *Obesity.* Edited by A. J. Stunkard. Philadelphia, W. B. Saunders, Co. 1980.

5

Practical Methods of Measuring Body Composition

Andrew S. Jackson

INTRODUCTION

Body composition is an important component of exercise prescription and health management programs. Many methods are
available for measuring body density. Laboratory methods
include underwater weighing, volume displacement, radiographic analysis, potassium-40, isotropic dilution, and ultrasound techniques [1]. These laboratory techniques are valid
but not practical for mass testing because they are time con-
suming and require considerable equipment, space, and trained
technicians. A common field test of body composition is to use
anthropometric measurements such as skinfold fat, body circumferences, and body diameters. The anthropometric methods
are less valid but more practical for mass testing. Various

Copyright © 1984 by Spectrum Publications, Inc., *Evaluation and Treatment of Obesity*, edited by J. Storlie and H. A. Jordan.

combinations of anthropometric variables are combined into a multiple regression equation with a function to predict a criterion. Hydrostatically measured body density has been the laboratory criterion most often used.

Since the early 1950s researchers have published body density prediction equations and well over 100 different equations appear in the literature. The equations are termed either "population specific" or "generalized." Population specific equations have been developed with data from relatively homogeneous samples (e.g., college-age males or females). The more recent research method has been to develop generalized equations which have been developed on samples varying greatly in age and body fatness. The purposes of this chapter are to: (1) examine the development of body composition prediction equations, and (2) provide field methods that are valid and practical for use with adults.

HEIGHT–WEIGHT

The most common body composition method used by clinicians is to recommend a suitable weight for a given height, frame size, and sex. Height–weight indicies have a major limitation. Body weight is generally divided into three components: bone, muscle, and fat. Lean body mass is composed of the bone and muscle weight. A person is overweight if his body weight exceeds the value that is standard for a person of a given sex, height, and frame size. These standard weight norms are obtained from tables based on population averages. A major deficiency of the standard height and weight table is the inability to differentiate lean body mass from fat weight. Although a standard height–weight index has been widely used for determining overweight in patients, its utility for estimating fat proportions is limited. For example, most football players would be overweight according to the standard height–weight index, but their percent body fat tends to be average to low.

Skinfold fat and body circumferences are the anthropometric variables most commonly used in body density prediction equations. Provided in Table 1 are the standard errors of

Table 1. Linear Correlations and Standard Errors for Predicting Body Density and Percent Body Fat from Anthropometric Variables

Variable	Female sample (N=283)			Male sample (N=402)		
	r	SE(BD)	SE(Pct fat)	r	SE(BD)	SE(Pct fat)
Age	-0.35	0.015	6.7	-0.38	0.017	7.3
Height	-0.06	0.016	7.1	-0.03	0.018	7.9
Weight	-0.63	0.012	5.5	-0.63	0.014	6.1
Body mass index[a]	-0.70	0.011	5.1	-0.69	0.014	5.7
Sum of seven skinfolds	-0.83	0.009	4.0	-0.88	0.009	3.8
Waist girth	-0.71	0.011	5.0	-0.80	0.011	4.7
Gluteal girth	-0.74	0.010	4.8	-0.69	0.013	5.7
Thigh girth	-0.68	0.012	5.2	-0.64	0.014	6.1
Biceps girth	-0.63	0.012	5.5	-0.51	0.016	6.8

[a]Body mass index = wt/ht^2, where weight is in kilograms and height in meters.

prediction and linear correlations between selected anthropometric variables and hydrostatically measured body density.
The statistics were developed with large samples of men [2]
and women [3] who varied considerably in age and body composition. As these data show, body density is most highly correlated with the sum of seven skinfolds. These data show the
major advantage of using skinfolds, or body circumferences,
over height and weight. Body density can be predicted with
greater accuracy.

POPULATION SPECIFIC EQUATIONS

The first body composition regression equations using
anthropometric techniques were published in 1951 by Brozek
and Keys [4], who used skinfolds to estimate body density for
young and middle-aged men. In the early 1960s Sloan et al.
[5,6] and Young et al. [7-10] published similar equations for
women of selected age groups. These first prediction equations
were developed by using various combinations of skinfold measurements. From the middle 1960s to the 1970s numerous
researchers published additional equations for women and men.
A summary of these studies may be found in another source
[11]. The objective of the research was to produce more accurate prediction equations. In addition to skinfold measurements, several body circumferences and, in some instances,
bone diameters were used as independent variables. During this
era, electronic computers and stepwise multiple regression computer programs became readily available to researchers. This
increased computing capacity made it easy to analyze a large
number of variables and select the combination of anthropometric variables that produced the highest multiple correlation.
The equations consisting of skinfolds, circumferences, and
diameters were more accurate than the earlier equations that
used just skinfolds; this was especially true for women [12] and
middle-aged men [13].

Population specific equations have been developed on
samples of relatively homogeneous subjects and can only be

used with similar subjects. If population specific equations are to be used, it is important to select the appropriate equation. It was shown [14,15] that equations developed on college-age males overestimated the fatness of lean world class runners and underpredicted the body fatness of middle aged men. Using gender specific equations and applying them to the opposite sex produces a constant prediction error of about 0.025g/ml (11% fat).

GENERALIZED EQUATIONS

The more recent thinking has been to develop generalized rather than population specific equations. The specific equations provide valid estimates with subjects representative of the defined population, but the more specific the population, the less general application an equation will have. The approach taken in generalized studies was to use a sample representative of heterogeneous populations and develop a regression model to account for the important sources of variability of the heterogeneous population. Then one equation can be used where several population specific equations were needed.

The research on population specific equations provides the scientific foundation for the development of generalized equations. Linear regression models have been used to develop population specific equations. However, in heterogeneous populations, the relation between skinfold fat and body density is not linear. This is shown in Figure 1 and demonstrates that the use of a linear regression model will produce large prediction errors at the extremes of the bivariate distribution. Several investigators [2,3,16] have shown that equations are age specific. Durnin and Wormersly [16] were able to show that aging variation was due to differences in the intercept of the regression line rather than the slope. Intercept differences can be corrected by using statistically derived constants. Lastly, skinfold measurements tend to be highly correlated [17]; thus, the sum of several measurements provide a more reliable measure of total subcutaneous fat.

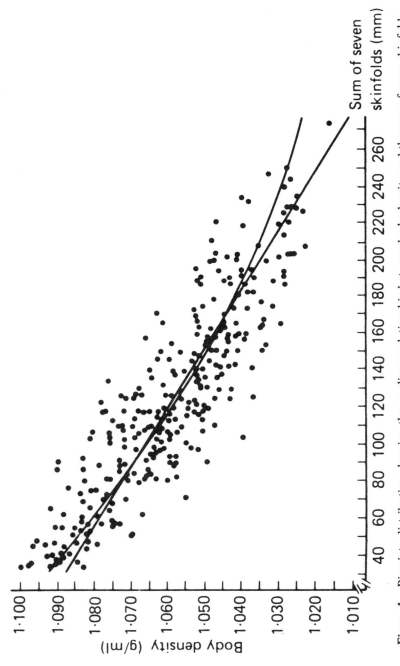

Figure 1. Bivariate distribution showing the nonlinear relationship between body density and the sum of seven skinfolds. From Baumgartner, T. A. and Jackson, A. S. *Measurement for Evaluation in Physical Education*. W. C. Brown, Dubuque, 1982, 2nd Ed., p. 292. Reprinted by permission of W. C. Brown Co., Dubuque.

Generalized body density prediction equations were developed for men [2] and women [3]. Provided in Table 2 are descriptive statistics on the subjects used in this research. Equations were developed with the sum of seven skinfolds and selected sum of three. The sums of three and seven skinfolds are highly correlated ($r \geq 0.97$), which shows that either sum could be used. Multivariate regression models consisting of the quadratic sum of skinfolds in combination with age were developed to account for the non-linear relationship (Figure 1) and aging. These generalized equations can be found in other sources [2,3,11,18]. The equations for the sum of three skinfolds are reproduced at the bottom of Tables 4 and 5. Furnished in Table 3 are the statistics supporting the validity of the generalized equations. Provided are the correlations and standard errors obtained on the samples used to develop and cross-validate the equations. These statistics are within the ranges reported by researchers who published population specific equations. The cross-validation statistics are nearly identical to the original regression statistics and provide the strongest evidence supporting the validity of the generalized equations. Additionally, the generalized equations' accuracy were found to be consistent over these variable groupings of subjects. These data show that one generalized equation can be used with the accuracy obtained with several population specific equations. The generalized approach provides clinicians with equations that can be used to measure the body composition of most adults without regard for age and body fatness.

Suggested Methods

Age and the sum of three skinfolds are needed to evaluate an adult's body composition. Two different sums of three skinfolds are recommended for men and women. The preferred sum of three skinfolds are; for MEN, sum of *chest, abdomen* and *thigh* skinfolds; for WOMEN, sum of *triceps, suprailium,* and *thigh* skinfolds. These different sums were selected because they provide a good representation of the total body and were highly correlated with the sum of seven skinfolds.

Table 2. Descriptive Statistics for Anthropometric Variables

Variable	Adult males (N=402)			Adult females (N=283)		
	Mean	SD	Range	Mean	SD	Range
General characteristics						
Age (yrs)	32.8	11.0	18–61	31.8	11.5	18–55
Height (cm)	179.0	6.4	163–201	168.6	5.8	152–185
Weight (kg)	78.2	11.7	53–123	57.5	7.4	36–88
Body mass index (wt/ht)	24.4	3.2	17–37	20.2	2.2	14–31
Laboratory determined						
Body density (g/ml)	1.058	0.018	1.016–1.100	1.044	0.016	1.002–1.091
Percent fat (%)	17.9	8.0	1–37	24.4	7.2	8–44
Lean weight (kg)	63.5	7.3	47–100	43.1	4.2	30–54
Fat weight (kg)	14.6	7.9	1–42	14.3	5.7	2–35
Skinfolds (mm)						
Chest	15.2	8.0	3–41	12.6	4.8	3–26
Axilla	17.3	8.7	4–39	13.0	6.1	3–33
Triceps	14.2	6.1	3–31	18.2	5.9	5–41
Subscapula	16.0	7.0	5–45	14.2	6.4	5–41
Abdomen	25.1	10.8	5–56	24.2	9.6	4–36
Suprailium	16.2	8.9	3–53	14.0	7.1	3–40
Thigh	18.9	7.7	4–48	29.5	8.0	7–53
Sum of skinfolds (mm)						
Sum of seven	122.9	52.0	31–272	125.6	42.0	35–266
Sum of three[a]	59.2	24.5	10–118	61.6	19.0	16–126

[a] Sum of three: In men, chest, abdomen, and thigh skinfolds. In women, triceps, suprailium, and thigh skinfolds.

Table 3. Validation and Cross-Validation Statistics of Generalized Equations

	Validation study			Cross-validation study		
Equation[a]	N	R	SE	N	R	SE
Male sample (2)						
E7, E7^2, age	308	0.902	0.0078	95	0.915	0.0078
E3, E7^2, age	308	0.905	0.0072	95	0.917	0.0077
Female sample (3)						
E7, E7^2, age	249	0.852	0.0083	82	0.803	0.0085
E3, E3^2, age	249	0.842	0.0087	82	0.820	0.0081

[a]In each case, E is the sum of three skinfolds. In males, chest, abdomen, and thigh; in females, triceps, suprailium, and thigh.

The accuracy of body density estimates from regression equations is dependent upon securing accurate measures of skinfold fat. Accuracy is enhanced by using a suitable caliper and having a trained technician measure skinfold fat at the proper location. For the development of the generalized equations, all measurements were taken on the right side of the body with a calibrated skinfold caliper (Lange caliper) which had a constant pressure of 10 g/mm². The skinfold sites used for the sum of three equations are described below. Pictures are provided to help standardize methods.

1. *Chest*: (Figure 2) A diagonal fold taken one half of the distance between the anterior axillary line and nipple. The site is used for men.

2. *Abdominal*: A vertical fold taken at a lateral distance of approximately 2 cm from the umbilicus (Figure 3). The site is used for men.

3. *Thigh*: A vertical fold on the anterior aspect of the thigh, midway between hip and knee joints (Figure 4). This site used for both men and women's equations.

4. *Triceps*: A vertical fold on the posterior midline of the upper arm (over triceps muscle), halfway between the acromion and olecranon processes; the elbow should be extended and relaxed (Figure 5). This site is used in the women's equation.

5. *Suprailium*: A diagonal fold above the crest of the ilium at the spot where an imaginary line would come down from the anterior axillary line (Figure 6). This site is used in the women's equation.

The skinfold is grasped firmly by the thumb and index finger; the caliper is perpendicular to the fold at approximately 1 cm (¼ in.) from the thumb and finger. Then the caliper grip is released so that full tension is exerted on the skinfold. In grasping the skinfold, the pads at the tip of thumb and finger are used. Female testers normally need to trim their nails. The dial is read to the nearest 0.5 mm approximately 1 to 2 seconds after the grip has been released. A minimum of two measurements should be taken at each site. If the repeated measurement

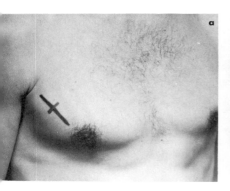
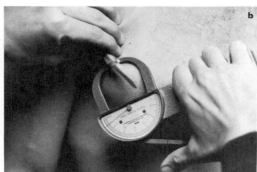

Figure 2. Test site (a) and placement of calipers for chest skinfold (b).

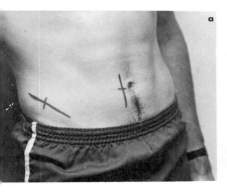
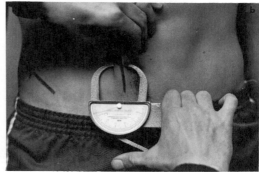

Figure 3. Test site (a) and placement of calipers for abdominal skinfold (b).

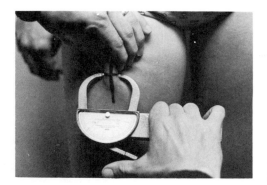

Figure 4. Caliper placement for thigh skinfold.

a

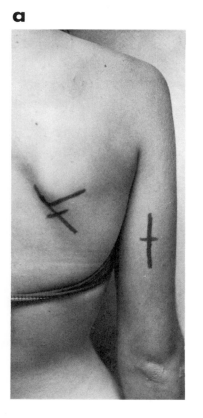

b

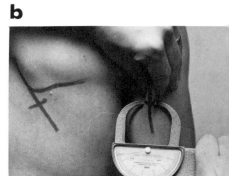

Figure 5. Test site (a) and
placement of calipers for
triceps skinfold (b).

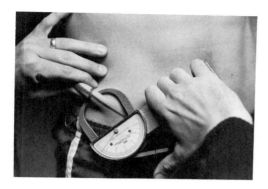

Figure 6. Placement of calipers for suprailium skinfold. Test site is shown in Figure 3 (a).

varies by more than 1 mm, a third should be taken. If consecutive fat measurements become smaller and smaller, the fat is being compressed; this occurs mainly with "fleshy" people. The tester should go on to the next site and return to the trouble spot after finishing the other measurements; the final value will be the average of the two that seem to best represent the skinfold fat site. It is better to take measurements when the skin is dry because when the skin is moist or wet the tester may grasp extra skin (fat) and get larger values. Practice is necessary to insure consistent results. Accuracy can be insured by having several technicians take the same measurements and comparing results. Numerous calipers are presently available, but in our judgment, it is desirable to have a caliper with a constant pressure of 10 g/mm². Some of the new inexpensive calipers do not have a constant pressure and, with untrained testers, the errors can be quite large.

The calculations can be somewhat difficult to complete by hand. Tables 4 and 5 are provided to expedite the calculation of percent body fat from the sum of three skinfolds and age. The tables were computer generated using the generalized body density equations which are provided at the bottom of the tables. Many labs have access to microcomputers which can be programmed to make the necessary calculations.

Table 4.   Percent Fat Estimates for Men: Sum of Chest, Abdominal and Thigh Skinfolds

Sum of skinfolds (mm)	Age to the last year								
	Under 22	to 27	23 to 32	28 to 37	33 to 42	38 to 47	48 to 52	53 to 57	Over 58
8–10	1.3	1.8	2.3	2.9	3.4	3.9	4.5	5.0	5.5
11–13	2.2	2.8	3.3	3.9	4.4	4.9	5.5	6.0	6.5
14–16	3.2	3.8	4.3	4.8	5.4	5.9	6.4	7.0	7.5
17–19	4.2	4.7	5.3	5.8	6.3	6.9	7.4	8.0	8.5
20–22	5.1	5.7	6.2	6.8	7.3	7.9	8.4	8.9	9.5
23–25	6.1	6.6	7.2	7.7	8.3	8.8	9.4	9.9	10.5
26–28	7.0	7.6	8.1	8.7	9.2	9.8	10.3	10.9	11.4
29–31	8.0	8.5	9.1	9.6	10.2	10.7	11.3	11.8	12.4
32–34	8.9	9.4	10.0	10.5	11.1	11.6	12.2	12.8	13.3
35–37	9.8	10.4	10.9	11.5	12.0	12.6	13.1	13.7	14.3
38–40	10.7	11.3	11.8	12.4	12.9	13.5	14.1	14.6	15.2
41–43	11.6	12.2	12.7	13.3	13.8	14.4	15.0	15.5	16.1
44–46	12.5	13.1	13.6	14.2	14.7	15.3	15.9	16.4	17.0
47–49	13.4	13.9	14.5	15.1	15.6	16.2	16.8	17.3	17.9
50–52	14.3	14.8	15.4	15.9	16.5	17.1	17.6	18.2	18.8
53–55	15.1	15.7	16.2	16.8	17.4	17.9	18.5	18.1	19.7
56–58	16.0	16.5	17.1	17.7	18.2	18.8	19.4	20.0	20.5
59–61	16.9	17.4	17.9	18.5	19.1	19.7	20.2	20.8	21.4
62–64	17.6	18.2	18.8	19.4	19.9	20.5	21.1	21.7	22.2
65–67	18.5	19.0	19.6	20.2	20.8	21.3	21.9	22.5	23.1

Sum of Skinfolds									
68–70	19.3	19.9	20.4	21.0	21.6	22.2	22.7	23.3	23.9
71–73	20.1	20.7	21.2	21.8	22.4	23.0	23.6	24.1	24.7
74–76	20.9	21.5	22.0	22.6	23.2	23.8	24.4	25.0	25.5
77–79	21.7	22.2	22.8	23.4	24.0	24.6	25.2	25.8	26.3
80–82	22.4	23.0	23.6	24.2	24.8	25.4	25.9	26.5	27.1
83–85	23.2	23.8	24.4	25.0	25.5	26.1	26.7	27.3	27.9
86–88	24.0	24.5	25.1	25.7	26.3	26.9	27.5	28.1	28.7
89–91	24.7	25.3	25.9	26.5	27.1	27.6	28.2	28.8	29.4
92–94	25.4	26.0	26.6	27.2	27.8	28.4	29.0	29.6	30.2
95–97	26.1	16.7	27.3	27.9	28.5	29.1	29.7	30.3	30.9
98–100	26.9	27.4	28.0	28.6	29.2	29.8	30.4	31.0	31.6
101–103	27.5	28.1	28.7	29.3	29.9	30.5	31.1	31.7	32.3
104–106	28.2	28.8	29.4	30.0	30.6	31.2	31.8	32.4	33.0
107–109	28.9	29.5	30.1	30.7	31.3	31.9	32.5	33.1	33.7
110–112	29.6	30.2	30.8	31.4	32.0	32.6	33.2	33.8	34.4
113–115	30.2	30.8	31.4	32.0	32.6	33.2	33.8	34.5	35.1
116–118	30.9	31.5	32.1	32.7	33.3	33.9	34.5	35.1	35.7
119–121	31.5	32.1	32.7	33.3	33.9	34.5	35.1	35.7	36.4
122–124	32.1	32.7	33.3	33.9	34.5	35.1	35.8	36.4	37.0
125–127	32.7	33.3	33.9	34.5	35.1	35.8	36.4	37.0	37.6

$BD = 1.1093800 - 0.0008267(X_1) + 0.0000016(X_1)^2 - 0.00002574(X_2)$, where X_1 is sum of chest, abdominal and thigh skinfolds and X_2 is age in years. Percent fat $= (495/BD) - 450$.

From Baumgartner, T. A., and Jackson, A. S. *Measurement for Evaluation in Physical Education.* W. C. Brown, Dubuque, 1982, 2nd Ed., p. 295. Reprinted by permission of W. C. Brown Co., Dubuque.

Table 5. Percent Fat Estimates for Women: Sum Triceps, Suprailium and Thigh Skinfolds

Sum of skinfolds (mm)	Age to the last year								
	Under 22	23 to 27	28 to 32	33 to 37	38 to 42	43 to 47	48 to 52	53 to 57	Over 58
23–25	9.7	9.9	10.2	10.4	10.7	10.9	11.2	11.4	11.7
26–28	11.0	11.2	11.5	11.7	12.0	12.3	12.5	12.7	13.0
29–31	12.3	12.5	12.8	13.0	13.3	13.5	13.8	14.0	14.3
32–34	13.6	13.8	14.0	14.3	14.5	14.8	15.0	15.3	15.5
35–37	14.8	15.0	15.3	15.5	15.8	16.0	16.3	16.5	16.8
38–40	16.0	16.3	16.5	16.7	17.0	17.2	17.5	17.7	18.0
41–43	17.2	17.4	17.7	17.9	18.2	18.4	18.7	18.9	19.2
44–46	18.3	18.6	18.8	19.1	19.3	19.6	19.8	20.1	20.3
47–49	19.5	19.7	20.0	20.2	20.5	20.7	21.0	21.2	21.5
50–52	20.6	20.8	21.1	21.3	21.6	21.8	22.1	22.3	22.6
53–55	21.7	21.9	22.1	22.4	22.6	22.9	23.1	23.4	23.6
56–58	22.7	23.0	23.2	23.4	23.7	23.9	24.2	24.4	24.7
59–61	23.7	24.0	24.2	24.5	24.7	25.0	25.2	25.5	25.7
62–64	24.7	25.0	25.2	25.5	35.7	26.0	26.7	26.4	26.7

65–67	25.7	25.9	26.2	26.4	26.7	26.9	27.2	27.4	27.7
68–70	26.6	26.9	27.1	27.4	27.6	27.9	28.1	28.4	28.6
71–73	27.5	27.8	28.0	28.3	28.5	28.8	29.0	29.3	29.5
74–76	28.4	28.7	28.9	29.2	29.4	29.7	29.9	30.2	30.4
77–79	29.3	29.5	29.8	30.0	30.3	30.5	30.8	31.0	31.3
80–82	30.1	30.4	30.6	30.9	31.1	31.4	31.6	31.9	32.1
83–85	30.9	31.2	31.4	31.7	31.9	32.2	32.4	32.7	32.9
86–88	31.7	32.0	32.2	32.5	32.7	32.9	33.2	33.4	33.7
89–91	32.5	32.7	33.0	33.2	33.5	33.7	33.9	34.2	34.4
92–94	33.2	33.4	33.7	33.9	34.2	34.4	34.7	34.9	35.2
95–97	33.9	34.1	34.4	34.6	34.9	35.1	35.4	35.6	35.9
98–100	34.6	34.8	35.1	35.3	35.5	35.8	36.0	36.3	36.5
101–103	35.3	35.4	35.7	35.9	36.2	36.4	36.7	36.9	37.2
104–106	35.8	36.1	36.3	36.6	36.8	37.1	37.3	37.5	37.8
107–109	36.4	36.7	36.9	37.1	37.4	37.6	37.9	38.1	38.4
110–112	37.0	37.2	37.5	37.7	38.0	38.2	38.5	38.7	38.9
113–115	37.5	37.8	38.0	38.2	38.5	38.7	39.0	39.2	39.5
116–118	38.0	38.3	38.5	38.8	39.0	39.3	39.5	39.7	40.0
119–121	38.5	38.7	39.0	39.2	39.5	39.7	40.0	40.2	40.5
122–124	39.0	39.2	39.4	39.7	39.9	40.2	40.4	40.7	40.9
125–127	39.4	39.6	39.9	40.1	40.4	40.6	40.9	41.1	41.4
128–130	39.8	40.0	40.3	40.5	40.8	41.0	41.3	41.5	41.8

BD = $1.0994921 - 0.0009929(X_1) + 0.0000023(X_1^2) - 0.0001392(X_2)$, where X_1 is the sum of triceps, suprailium and thigh skinfolds and X_2 is age in years.

From Baumgartner, T. A., and Jackson, A. S. *Measurement for Evaluation in Physical Education*. W. C. Brown, Dubuque, 1982, 2nd Ed., p. 296. Reprinted by permission of W. C. Brown Co., Dubuque.

INTERPRETATION

This chapter provides an overview of the research on the prediction of body density and the methods that are valid and practical for measuring the body composition of adults. But, what is an optional level of body fatness? This is difficult to determine with certainty; however, normative data has provided some guidelines. For satisfactory health levels, Lohman [20] suggests levels of 10% to 22% fat content in men and 20% to 32% fat content in women are considered suitable. For athletes, however, these levels would be too high. Wilmore [21] has published a comprehensive summary of data published with athletes. The average levels are about 12% for males and 18% for females. For athletes in events that place emphasis on efficient body movement (e.g., distance runner, football back, gymnast, etc.), the body fat levels tend to range from 4% to 10% for males and 13% to 18% for females.

Extremely low body fat levels can have a negative effect on health and physical performance. For this reason, fat content levels ranging from 3% to 7% and 10% to 20% should be considered minimal levels for men and women respectively.

REFERENCES

1. Behnke, A. R., and Wilmore, J. H. *Evaluation and Regulation of Body Build and Composition.* Englewood Cliffs; Prentice Hall, Inc., 1974.
2. Jackson, A. S., and Pollock, M. L. Generalized equations for predicting body density of men. *Br. J. Nutr. 40*:497-504, 1978.
3. Jackson, A. S., Pollock, M. L., and Ward, A. Generalized equations for predicting body density of women. *Med. Sci. in Sports and Exercise 12*:175-182, 1980.
4. Brozek, J., and Keys, A. The evaluation of leanness-fatness in man: norms and intercorrelations. *Br. J. Nutr. 5*:194-206, 1951.
5. Sloan, A. W. Estimation of body fat in young men. *J. Appl. Physiol. 23*:311-315, 1967.
6. Sloan, A. W., Burt, J. J., and Blyth, C. S. Estimation of body fat in young women. *J. Appl. Physiol. 17*:967-970, 1962.
7. Young, C. M. Prediction of specific gravity and body fatness in older women. *J. Am. Dietet. Assoc. 45*:333-338, 1964.

8. Young, C. M., Blondin, J., Tensuan, R., and Fryer, J. Body composition studies of "older" women thirty to seventy years of age. *Ann. N.Y. Acad. Sci. 110*:589-607, 1963.
9. Young, C. M., Martin, J., Chihan, M., McCarthy, M., Manniello, M. J., Harmuth, E. H., and Fryer, J. H. Body composition of young women. *J. Am. Dietet. Assoc. 38*:332-340, 1961.
10. Young, C. M., Martin, M., Tensuan, R., and Blondin, J. Predicting specific gravity and body fatness in young women. *J. Am. Dietet. Assoc. 40*:102-107, 1962.
11. Baumgartner, T. A., and Jackson, A. S. Chapter 7: Evaluating physical fitness. In *Measurement for Evaluation in Physical Education.* Dubuque, Wm. C. Brown Co., 1982, 2nd edition.
12. Pollock, M. L., Laughridge, E., Coleman, B., Linnerud, A. C., and Jackson, A. S. Prediction body density in young and middle-aged women. *J. Appl. Physiol. 38*:745-749, 1975.
13. Pollock, M. L., Hickman, T., Kendrick, A., et al: Prediction of body density in young and middle-aged men. *J. Appl. Physiol. 40*:300-304, 1976.
14. Pollock, M. L., Jackson, A. S., Ayres, J., Ward, A., Linnerud, A., and Gettman, L. Body composition of elite class distance runners. *Ann. N.Y. Acad. Sci. 301*:361-370, 1977.
15. Jackson, A. S., and Pollock, M. L. Prediction accuracy of body density, lean and body weight, and total body volume equations. *Med. Sci. Sports 9*:197-201, 1977.
16. Durnin, J. F. G. A., and Wormersley, J. Body fat assessed from total body density and its estimation from skinfold thickness; measurements on 481 men and women aged from 16 to 72 years. *Br. J. Nutr. 32*:77-92, 1974.
17. Jackson, A. S., and Pollock, M. L. Factor analysis and multivariate scaling of anthropometric variables for the assessment of body composition. *Med. Sci. Sports 8*:196-203, 1976.
18. Pollock, M. L., Schmidt, D. H., and Jackson, A. S. Measurement of cardiorespiratory fitness and body composition in the clinical setting. *Comp. Therapy 6*:12-27, 1980.
19. Siri, W. E. Body composition from fluid spaces and density. In *Techniques for Measuring Body Composition.* Ed. by J. Brozek and A. Hanschel, pp. 223-224. Washington, D.C., National Academy of Science, 1961.
20. Lohman, T. G. Body composition in sports medicine. *Phys. Sports Med. 10*:46-58, 1982.
21. Wilmore, J. H. *Training for Sport and Activity: The Physiological Basis of the Conditioning Process.* Boston, Allyn and Bacon, 1982, 2nd edition.

Psychological Factors Related to Eating and Activity Behaviors

Jean Storlie

INTRODUCTION

Effective design and evaluation of obesity treatment programs that focus on behavioral and lifestyle change requires an understanding of related psychological factors. Several psychosocial issues appear to have etiological significance in obesity; however, the extent to which each of these factors contributes to the state of obesity of a given individual is variable [1–4]. It is, therefore, critical to identify the underlying causes of obesity on an individual basis, develop appropriate treatment goals, and monitor change throughout the course of treatment. Unfortunately, simple straightforward procedures are not available to objectively and systematically evaluate the obese person from a psychological viewpoint.

Psychological assessment of obesity is complicated. In the first place, human beings are extremely complex and individual

Copyright © 1984 by Spectrum Publications, Inc., *Evaluation and Treatment of Obesity*, edited by J. Storlie and H. A. Jordan.

creatures. Obesity is influenced by numerous interrelated factors, both psychological and biological in nature [5]; these factors are often difficult to isolate and quantify. Since behaviors are interdependent with cognitions, affect, and social circumstances specific to each individual, effective assessment must also consider these factors [4]. Furthermore, assessment procedures are complicated by the subjective nature of self-reporting devices.

Over the years, considerable attention has been given to psychological appraisal of obesity. Early work focused primarily on the question: How does the psychological make-up of the obese person differ from normal-weight people? The following standardized psychological tools have been applied to the assessment of obese individuals: MMPI [6–8], SCL-90 [6,9,10], Rorschach Test [11], Bell Adjustment Inventory [12,13], 16 Personality Factor Questionnaire [14], Cattel Neuroticism Scale [14], and Nowlis Mood Checklist [15]. These investigations have contributed to the identification of critical psychological issues in obesity.

Although certain tendencies were revealed, it has since become apparent that obese individuals do not share a "typical" personality or behavioral structure [3,8]. For example, Grinker [15] found that juvenile-onset obesity was associated with greater disturbances in body image. Further, these individuals responded better to psychotherapy, while those with adult-onset obesity experienced better results with nutrition and behavioral education. Schumaker et al. [16] characterized two obese eating styles and demonstrated that different therapies were more effective with each style. These results validate the conclusion that obesity is a complex syndrome affecting a diverse group of people and requiring varied intervention techniques [3]. A thorough evaluation process is recommended to pair appropriate treatment strategies with individuals [3,4,17].

The evaluation process should include: (1) medical status, (2) weight history, (3) family and socio-economic situation, (4) psychological history and functioning, (5) emotional and cognitive structure, and (6) behavioral profile [4,17]. To date, an objective, comprehensive, and standardized assessment device

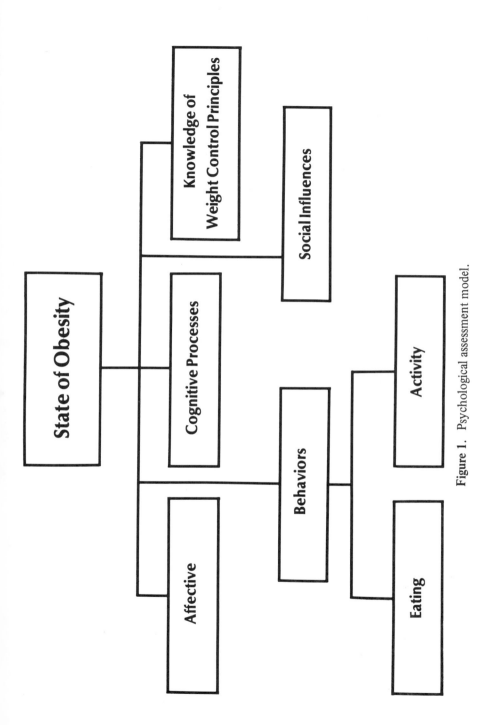

Figure 1. Psychological assessment model.

to cover these issues has not been constructed and validated. A compilation of assessment tools could be utilized to evaluate these factors, although this presents a problem in terms of efficiency and time.

Considering the state of the art, this chapter is intended to address issues pertinent to the assessment of weight-related behaviors. Discussion focuses on the scope, content, and rationale for comprehensive psychological assessment of obesity. A theoretical model for approaching the assessment process (Figure 1) is introduced and five major categories will be considered: (1) knowledge of weight control principles, (2) cognitive processes, (3) affect, (4) social influences, and (5) weight-related behaviors.

KNOWLEDGE OF WEIGHT CONTROL PRINCIPLES

Assessing an individual's knowledge of weight control principles is, perhaps, the least complicated aspect of the assessment process. In fact, if inappropriate behaviors result from a lack of information, the intervention process is also simplified. Unfortunately, in most cases the individual is well aware of the facts and information, yet does not behave accordingly. It is not uncommon to find clients who know as much, if not more about calories in food than dietitians. In these circumstances, a significantly different intervention process is required than for the person who simply lacks appropriate knowledge.

Establishing the baseline level of knowledge prior to implementing any treatment is valuable for the following reasons:

1. To design the education program so the current knowledge base will facilitate the ability to make informed choices and positive behavior changes.
2. To determine if lack of knowledge is limiting change or if the problem lies elsewhere.
3. To evaluate how effectively the educational processes impact the participants' level of knowledge.

Most assessment devices include some questions related to knowledge. The Master Questionnaire, developed by Margaret Straw [18], includes 62 true–false questions relating to knowledge. Marston [3] developed a Knowledge Test© which is used in his correspondence weight reduction program. Although these questionnaires are helpful for assessing knowledge, it may be necessary to develop tests specific to the program being evaluated, since the educational content tends to vary slightly from program to program.

When developing a knowledge test for purposes of evaluating treatment effectiveness, it is important that the content of the test relate directly to the learning objectives. Further, an attempt should be made to prioritize the information, separating: What is *essential* knowledge? What is *worthwhile* knowledge? What is *interesting* knowledge? Although the education program should still include interesting and worthwhile information, it is beneficial to isolate the most significant facts and figures for assessment purposes. Keep in mind what participants need to know in order to make informed choices and change behavior accordingly.

Table 1 lists several questions related to the major concepts of weight control (i.e., energy balance, ideal weight, weight loss

Table 1.   Questions to Test Knowledge of Weight Control Principles

How does energy balance regulate body weight?

How many calories are in one pound of body fat?

What is a safe and appropriate rate of weight loss?

How many calories are burned in certain types of exercise?

Calorically, how do food and exercise relate? (e.g., how many miles do you need to walk to burn off an order of french fries?)

Why is percentage of body fat more appropriate than height/weight determination of ideal weight?

Table 2.   Questions to Test Knowledge of Exercise and Fitness

What types of exercise burn calories? How much is needed? How often should a person exercise?

What is appropriate clothing and footwear for specific exercises?

What characterizes a good fitness program? How do the different forms of exercise (strength, flexibility and aerobic) benefit?

Why is exercise beneficial for weight control?

How does one monitor the intensity of exercise to remain within safe limits, yet improve fitness?

What is the minimum length of time for an exercise session in order to be effective?

How can injuries be prevented?

---

patterns). These questions are worded in general, open-ended terms to use as a guideline for appraising knowledge of weight control information. The format of questions should be determined according to the needs of the setting (method of scoring, population served, etc.).

Fitness concepts relating to the proper amount and type of exercise for weight control are also an important component of the educational process, particularly since there is a lot of misunderstanding in this area. Table 2 outlines questions which guide the process of assessing knowledge of fitness principles. It is important for adults beginning an exercise program to have a thorough understanding of knowledge in this area to manage their own fitness program safely and effectively.

The area of nutrition and dieting is flooded with misinformation. In fact, it is probable that the most readily available food in this country is not nutritious, and the most readily available nutrition information fallacious. This situation presents a challenge to the therapist intervening with nutrition education because overweight individuals are typically saturated with nutrition knowledge, some of it sound and some of it erroneous.

Table 3. Questions to Test Knowledge of Nutrition and Dieting

How do protein, fat and carbohydrates function in the body?

What is a good distribution of protein, fat, and carbohydrate?

What are the harmful and potentially dangerous effects of carbohydrate restriction and starvation?

Why are excessive amounts of protein and fat harmful?

What are the characteristics of a good diet for weight control?

What happens to the diet when certain food groups are eliminated?

Are vitamin supplements required during weight loss?

Which popular diets are potentially dangerous? Why? How can a diet be evaluated?

What are some nutrition recommendations for the American public to improve health?

Where are calories hidden in foods?

Further, the knowledge they have is believed to be true and accurate. Assessment of nutrition knowledge is, therefore, critical in beginning treatment. Table 3 presents questions which relate to specific aspects of these major concepts: (1) balanced diet, (2) starvation and ketosis, (3) vitamin supplementation, (4) evaluating popular diets, (5) nutrition goals for health, and (6) calories in foods/food groups. Misinformation often interferes with an individual's understanding of these concepts.

Other relevant information may be covered in the nutrition education process. For example, shopping and cooking techniques, planning menus, eating out, and handling special situations are important skills for managing caloric intake. Certain information is required to implement these skills. This information may be included in the evaluation process, either as "knowledge" or in reference to the actual behavior changes resulting from this information.

COGNITIVE PROCESSES

Individual interpretation of events has a direct impact on both emotions and behavior. To illustrate this point, imagine yourself walking down a street at night, and you hear footsteps approaching from behind. If the situation is interpreted with the thought "maybe it's a mugger," the emotional response will be fear and the resulting behavior will probably be either to fight or flight. If the same circumstance is interpreted, "it's just someone jogging," both the emotional and behavioral reactions will be quite different.

Cognitive processes, and thus interpretations of statements and events, are influenced by many factors. Past experience, social systems, and the environment all affect a person's cognitions. If the situation just described would happen to a person who has been raped, or to someone who has just been warned about the dangers of walking alone at night, or if the event occurred in a high crime neighborhood, the interpretation would be highly influenced. From this illustration, it is clear that the individual attitudes, values, and beliefs affect how each person interprets the world and, ultimately, behaves. The following discussion will focus on the cognitive issues which affect the ability to self-direct behavior.

Locus of Control

Rotter [19] introduced the locus of control construct, which is an attempt to classify one's beliefs about the relationship between a behavior and its outcome. Individuals with an external locus of control have generalized expectancies that events in their lives are controlled by factors over which they have little control (fate, luck, chance or other people who are more powerful than them). In contrast, others tend to believe that events in their lives result from their own behavior; this view is termed internal locus of control. O'Bryan [20] found that internally controlled individuals were more likely to engage in behavior that facilitates weight control.

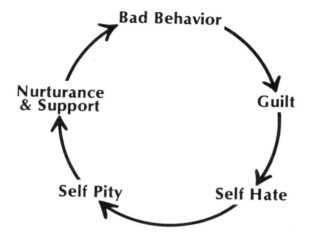

Figure 2. Self-defeating behavior cycle.

The idea that self control, or more specifically an internal locus of control, influences weight behaviors warrants discussion. Figure 2 illustrates how an event is linked to a corresponding cognitive interpretation, emotional response and loss of control. This Self-Defeating Behavior Cycle diagrams the justification for continuing the behavior.

Assume a person just ate a hot fudge sundae, interpreting this behavior (event) as "bad" due to past experiences and social pressure. The resulting emotions are guilt and self hate. After a process of self-flagellation with thoughts like, "I'm such a lousy person, I didn't mean to eat that sundae," the individual has difficulty accepting the behavior as within his/her realm of control. At this point, responsibility for the behavior is transferred to the outer world. The individual has punished him/herself, and experiences a sense of self pity. Thoughts like, "I can't help it . . . It's not my fault . . . If only . . .," begin to dominate the interpretation process. It is clear that the individual is now operating in an external locus and no longer believes in self control. The need for external support and reinforcement often leads back to eating, and "bad" behavior.

Table 4. Weight Locus of Control Scale

	Strongly disagree	Mildly disagree	Mildy agree	Strongly agree
1. Overweight problems are mainly a result of hereditary or physiological factors.	——	——	——	——
2. Overweight people need some tangible external motivation in order to reduce.	——	——	——	——
3. In overweight people, hunger is caused by the expectation of being hungry.	——	——	——	——
4. Overweight problems can be traced to poor eating habits which are relatively simple to change.	——	——	——	——
5. Overweight problems are mainly a result of lack of self-control.	——	——	——	——
6. Diet pills can be a valuable aid in weight reduction.	——	——	——	——
7. In overweight people, hunger is caused by stomach contractions and low blood sugar levels.	——	——	——	——
8. Overweight people will lose weight only when they can generate enough internal motivation.	——	——	——	——
9. A person who loses weight with diet pills will gain the weight back eventually.	——	——	——	——
10. Overweight problems can be traced to early childhood and are very resistant to change.	——	——	——	——

11. People who exercise today, do so only because everyone else is exercising.

12. If I exercise regularly, I can stay healthier.

13. If I am in poor physical condition it is because I have not been very active.

14. Staying in shape is largely a matter of being lucky enough to have the health it takes to be active.

15. No matter how hard I try, I will never be able to achieve a high level of fitness.

16. When I get tired easy or am short of breath, I know it is because I have not done what is necessary to stay fit.

17. People who are in good shape were fortunate enough to be naturally endowed with sound bodies.

18. Exercise could be hazardous because there are so many things which can go wrong with the body.

19. Being unfit is often the result of being too lazy to be active.

20. I can be active if I want to be regardless of the circumstances.

Items 1–10 from Tobias, L. L., and McDonald, M. L. Internal locus of control and weight loss: an insufficient condition. *Journal of Consulting and Clinical Psychology* 45:647–653, 1977. Items 11–16 from Langley, T. Relationship between success in a weight loss fitness program and locus of control reinforcement. Doctoral Dissertation, University of South Carolina, 1983.

It is possible that overeating stems from a predominantly external locus, but the Self-Defeating Behavior Cycle (Figure 2) may be entered at any phase. A person could function internally on the job, in the parent role, or other aspects of his/her life, but experience guilt when eating and end up losing control (i.e., enter the Self-Defeating Behavior Cycle). For this reason, Rotter's [21] classic locus of control scale has had inconsistent results in predicting success with weight control [22–24]. In fact, some researchers have concluded that locus of control is not a critical issue in weight control [25]. Others, however, proposed that a weight-related locus of control scale is required to verify this theory [26]. Table 4 presents a scale of this nature. Note that the items specifically apply to control of weight-related behaviors.

Assessment of weight-related locus of control can benefit the therapist in understanding each client's ability to "take charge," initiate change, and self-direct behavior. In cases where the weight-related locus is very external, the intervention process must either facilitate a shift in locus or externally manipulate behavior. A self-directed change process can be effective only if a person believes that he/she can control behavior. This issue may be so critical that therapists will need to consider developing both "internal" and "external" intervention plans to treat individuals according to their locus of control.

Irrational Beliefs

Albert Ellis [27] believes that certain thoughts cause emotional problems, creating and perpetuating self-defeating behavior. This philosophy has evolved into what is known as rational–emotive therapy (RET) [28]. Central to RET is the A–B–C Theory which links an activating event (A) to an emotional response (C) through a person's belief system (B). According to this theory, a person's belief system, rational or irrational, is responsible for the feelings that result from a set of circumstances. Emotional suffering and self-defeatist attitudes, therefore, stem from irrational beliefs.

Rational–emotive therapists attempt to restructure thinking by identifying and changing irrational beliefs that lead to inappropriate feelings [28]. Irrational beliefs generally take the form of self-talk with words like "should," "ought," and "must," (i.e., interpreting situations in absolute, unrealistic terms) that worry, preoccupy, and immobilize the person.

A perfect example of irrational thinking is when a person arrives at class and steps on the scale, saying "I had a bad week—I really blew it!" After discussing the events of the week, it turns out that one overeating episode occurred; however, the individual has interpreted it in absolute terms ("I blew the whole week," or "I am a failure").

The RET–ABC Model has many parallels to Rotter's locus of control construct. While both theories deal with cognitive influences, the emphasis in RET is on the emotional response to irrational beliefs and locus of control deals with the belief in self-directed behavior. These theories have clear application to weight control. Morelli [29] found that patients who failed to lose weight tend to engage in cognitive distortions, centered on asking "why" type questions. A self-defeatist attitude, which does not delineate constructive problem-solving techniques, results from these questions. Leon [30] linked self-control behaviors to cognitive processes enhancing decision-making and commitment. Foreyt [31] proposed that the following cognitions be assessed before initiating weight reduction: (1) perception of self-efficacy, (2) expectations for success, and (3) perception of efficacy of treatment. These guidelines, as well as the key phrases presented in Table 5, will facilitate the identification of irrational beliefs and cognitive distortions.

Rational interpretation of weight-related issues is exacerbated by the wealth of misinformation on diet and exercise that saturates our society. Greenberg et al. [2] described nutrition faddism as "America's favorite indoor sport," attributing the popularity of fad diets to promises of easy, effortless weight loss.* Since people believe this fallacious information to

---

*For a discussion of prevalent, erroneous beliefs about exercise, see B. A. Franklin, Exercise intervention for weight control: myths and misconceptions. In *Nutrition and Exercise in Obesity Management*, edited by J. Storlie and H. A. Jordan (New York, Spectrum Publications, 1984).

Table 5. Rational–Emotive Therapy

Concepts	Irrational Phrases
Worry-itis	What if . . .
Ownership vs. nonownership	I have to . . . I must . . . I should . . . You make me . . . I can't do it . . .
Awfulizing or catastrophizing	I'll never . . . . . . ever . . . . . . can't stand it . . . I *need* . . . It's terrible, awful All . . ., nothing
Self rejection	I'm just unlucky. I would be nothing without . . . Isn't that right?

be true, it clearly influences weight behaviors. Assessing an individual's belief in common myths and misconceptions (Table 6) will provide valuable insights into cognitions, emotions, locus of control, and behavior.

Values

Cognitive structure also consists of a person's values. Osman [32] constructed an entire weight reduction program on the premise that individual value systems dictate behavior and commitment to change. Obviously, if a person does not value exercise, it will not be a priority in his/her life, and will most likely *not* become a routine habit. Assessment of personal priorities and value systems is, therefore, worthwhile. Osman has developed several useful self-help tools that guide an individual into evaluating values related to weight control [32]. These tools could be incorporated into the assessment process. Another approach would be to have individuals indicate the importance

Table 6. Common Myths and Misconceptions

The only way to lose weight is to skip breakfast.

If I exercise, I'll get fat thighs.

I don't need exercise; I'm active all day.

I don't have time to exercise.

I gain five pounds just smelling food.

Bread and potatoes are fattening.

I'm addicted to sweets.

Obesity runs in my family.

My only pleasure is food.

I'm always hungry.

I have a cellulite problem.

Exercise causes bulky muscles.

I should lose five pounds a week.

It's natural to gain weight as you grow older.

of various aspects of their life on a Liekert scale. A few examples are listed below:

	Very little				Very much	
The time I spend with my family and friends	1	2	3	4	5	6
Performance in job/occupation	1	2	3	4	5	6
Maintaining my health	1	2	3	4	5	6
Pursuing an "optimal" level of health	1	2	3	4	5	6
Eating a healthy diet	1	2	3	4	5	6
Controlling weight	1	2	3	4	5	6
Engaging in regular exercise	1	2	3	4	5	6
Appearance and dress	1	2	3	4	5	6

As personal values are appraised, it is important to relate this information to the other cognitive processes. Values, attitudes, and beliefs interdependently affect emotions and behaviors.

AFFECT

The preceding discussion connected cognitions and affect with behavior. Clearly, these processes are intertwined and difficult to isolate. Thorough assessment of each area facilitates understanding the dynamics of individual functioning.

In 1955, Summerskill and Darling [33] found that obesity can be associated with varying states of emotional adjustment, from essentially normal to seriously disturbed. Further, when signs of good emotional adjustment are present it was felt that the chances of success with dieting are four times as great. In cases where poor emotional adjustment was evident, undesirable outcomes from dieting were noted. These early observations indicated need for thorough screening before initiating treatment.

Gold [34] discussed the following theories related to the emotional adjustment of the obese:

1. Oral activity is an adaption for coping with anxiety, tension, sorrow and frustration.
2. Hunger replaces feelings of excitement, sadness, or anger.
3. Food becomes a "drug" to cope with lack of social adjustment.
4. Hostility or resentment is reflected in poorly controlled, outwardly directed aggressive impulses.

Obese individuals have been characterized as more troubled, tense, frustrated, driven, overwrought, and submissive [14]. They tend to exhibit symptoms of increased anxiety, pain, repression, and defensiveness [11]. Low self esteem, body image disturbances, lack of interest in people, and poor communication skills have also been identified [8,11].

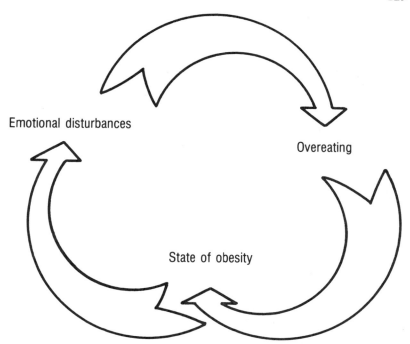

Emotional disturbances

Overeating

State of obesity

Figure 3.   Emotions and eating.

Although these affective characteristics have been used to describe the obese population, it is important to realize that not all obese individuals manifest these disturbances [33]. Clearly, the state of obesity has certain psychosocial consequences and vice versa, however it is a gross overgeneralization to classify all obese as emotionally disturbed. The most important questions to ask in the assessment process are: (1) Does the individual have any emotional problems? (2) If so, do the emotional problems lead to overeating, or does the state of obesity create the emotional problems? Both the emotional precursors to and consequences of obesity need to be identified and separated (Figure 3).

Emotional states related to overeating are frequently misunderstood. This issue is disguised in the "willpower" question: "Why are the obese unmotivated *to change*?" Motivation to change (or the lack of it) is not the problem; more directly, the

Table 7. Motivators

Needs	Fears
Love and affection	The Unknown
Pleasure	Facing other problems
Social outlet	Self-exploration
Stress management	Change
Self-reward	Growth
	Relating to people differently

critical question is: "What motivates the individual *to maintain* his/her current behaviors and weight status?" That is, the therapist must explore what *needs* are being met by these behaviors and what *fears* the individual must face in abandoning the behaviors (Table 7).

A craving for love and affection is frequently a drive to eat inappropriately (i.e., either overeat or eat when not hungry). This probably grows out of the nurturing attention mothers provide as they feed their children. It may not be quite as apparent, but just being overweight serves a need for some individuals, primarily as an escape from dealing with other problems.

The following case clearly illustrates this point. A 35-year-old female, who is married with two children, enrolled in a behavioral weight control program to lose about 40 pounds. She demonstrated excellent compliance and success, losing 25 pounds, walking five miles a day, and following a balanced 1500 calorie diet. Two weeks after the end of the program, she called the instructor in a distressed and worried state, expressing that she could not identify with herself as a "thin" person. She said, "I've always been fat and don't know how people will react to me now. When going to parties, I felt no one would care to talk to me—I was just Jim's wife . . . maybe, I need to take a class or start reading books, so I'll have something interesting to say." This woman was expressing fear of the unknown, fear of being socially inadequate, and fear of self-exploration and growth. Although she had demonstrated the ability to change her overt behaviors and lose weight, she was afraid of exposing and facing some deeper issues. Unfortunately, she did not opt to continue in treatment at that time and regained the lost weight.

Obviously, these emotional issues must be confronted and resolved in the course of treatment or the long-term prognosis will be poor. Early identification of these signs is critical. Further, long-term follow-up is necessary, as most emotional problems are deep-rooted. It is also valuable to document change and verify progress, since weight loss may not occur during the early phases of treatment, but emotional adjustment may improve. In these circumstances, success should be redefined and the client reinforced, accordingly.

The emotional consequences of obesity also aggravate the causative factors and perpetuate the obese state. A lack of self confidence and self esteem leads to feelings of inadequacy, loss of control, and overeating; in turn, overeating and obesity deteriorate one's sense of self.

Leon and Chamberlain [25] found that normal weight subjects felt better after eating, while subjects who had been or were currently obese felt worse after eating. The obese subjects related the negative mood to anger and guilt from eating. Hewitt [36] concluded that a negative mood associated with eating would further the weight control problem.

The stigmatizing attitudes directed toward the obese in our society have been identified as a severe emotional consequence of obesity [37–39]. Kalisch [37] considered a change in self concept critical to maintaining weight loss. With adolescents, however, Allon [38] felt that the stigma of obesity could either help or hinder weight reduction efforts. Craft [39] proposed that the severity of body image disturbances is related to age of onset, presence of other emotional problems, and exposure to stigmatizing attitudes during the formative years. It was observed that adolescents and children are more deeply affected than adults.

The depression associated with dieting [40] is another emotional manifestation which will interfere with positive growth and emotional adjustment. Without these changes, weight loss efforts are undermined. It is apparent that affective functioning relative to obesity has a significant impact on social adjustment and self-directed behavior.

SOCIAL INFLUENCES

Since the obese live in a "fat world" and must learn a new lifestyle when attempting to lose weight, Tobias and Gordon [41] recommended that sociopsychological factors need to be assessed and monitored, as well as the usual physiological measures. Krantz [42] observed that the social pressures operating on the obese are important determinants of their eating behavior, identifying a "social suppression" effect related to self-consciousness when eating. On the other hand, Rosenthal and Marx [43] identified two groups of overeaters: the emotional eater and the social eater. They felt that each group demonstrates a different pattern of skill deficit and, consequently, they require different treatment approaches. Eating which occurs in social situations was associated with a lack of assertiveness skills, while eating alone in response to painful emotions was indicative of inadequate coping skills.

Hawkins [44] related low assertiveness to an external locus of control. Inadequate communication skills, therefore, may be a significant contributor to self-defeating behavior. An instrument, such as the scale developed by Galassi [45] for college students, could help determine the following:

1. The type of assertive responses the client fails to elicit.
2. The interpersonal situations in which appropriate assertiveness skills are not utilized.
3. Patient selection for intensive assertiveness training and measurement of change in the course of training.

If assertive skill deficit is identified as a link to external locus and self-defeating behavior during the assessment process, the individual should be referred to an assertiveness training program as an adjunct to the weight reduction program. This will be critical in facilitating the skill development required to initiate self-directed behavior change. To clarify this point, recognize the person who passively relates to others, feeling victimized when he/she interacts with people. These social contacts reinforce feelings of self pity and loss of control. As an entry into the self-defeating behavior cycle (Figure 2), passive behavior, then, leads to overeating, the "bad" behavior. Guilt and self hate take over to perpetuate this unhealthy behavior cycle.

Granat [46] discussed several family issues which contribute to obesity, and encouraged professionals to recognize the important role of the family. A deficient or unsatisfying marital relationship could manifest itself in a weight problem. Further, spouses may rationalize eating behavior by blaming their partner for the reason they go out to eat, snack in the evening, avoid exercise, or select high calorie foods. Parents influence their children's behavior through role modeling, as well as parent–child conflicts. Mothers frequently gain excessive weight during and after childbirth as they adjust to a new role and relationship. The family situation plays a significant role in a person's life, and can either support or undermine weight loss efforts. These factors should be assessed and managed throughout treatment.

Socioeconomic factors also appear to have an influence. Kohrs [47] estimated the prevalence of obesity in Missouri residents. The following trends were identified:

1. The proportion of overweight women was inversely related to income and education.
2. A higher incidence of overweight men occurred with lower income and higher education levels.
3. The proportion of obese men was greater in urban than in rural populations.

Certainly, socioeconomic background will also influence the appropriateness of various treatment options. For example, a fitness program, consisting of three to five exercise classes each week may be very inconvenient for rural dwellers residing a great distance from town. Cost factors will rule out many programs for the lower socioeconomic groups. Stage of the life-cycle, age of onset, and sex differences will present problems unique to each group. It is much easier to facilitate and direct discussions with a homogeneous group because the individuals can better relate to one another. Both the individuals and groups serviced should be assessed to determine these socioeconomic influences in designing appropriate treatment plans.

Lastly, consider the impact of the media, on both a national and community level, when evaluating the social conditions affecting eating and activity behaviors.* In summary, social influences on weight-related behavior include social adjustment, family interactions, interpersonal and communication skills, socioeconomic status, and the media.

WEIGHT-RELATED BEHAVIORS

At the foundation of behavioral intervention for obesity is the underlying assumption that behavior change will produce weight loss. Although some current evidence [48] suggests there is reason to question this assumption, a review of behavioral theories is warranted, beginning with a review of eating habits and activity behavioral analysis.

Eating Habits

Brownell [49] suggested that the following variables should be considered in assessing eating behavior: cue responsiveness, eating styles, food choices, and food preferences.

Schacter's classic theory [50] on external cue responsiveness, which was introduced in 1968, proposed that eating for the obese is largely determined by external cues, such as the time of day, taste of food, and setting. He further proposed that the internal cues of hunger and satiety are irrelevant to eating

---

*This powerful influence will be discussed in further detail in *Innovation in Obesity Program Development*, edited by J. Storlie and H. A. Jordan (New York, Spectrum Publications, 1985).

behavior. Additional investigations [51–56] tended to support this theory, leading to the following conclusions:

1. For the obese, eating is either triggered by psychic states, such as anxiety, fear, and loneliness, or external food-related cues [51].
2. Normal weight subjects with a history of obesity also exhibit a similar pattern of externally controlled, stimulus-bound behavior [53].
3. Time has a greater influence on overweight individuals during the weekdays when their schedule is routine [54].

In 1973, Singh [57] showed that obese subjects responded more to emotional stimuli. This evidence could not be explained by Schacter's theory. Triggered by these questions, Wagner and Schumaker [58] conducted an investigation to determine the relationship between the external-cue theory and age of onset. The results demonstrated that the early-onset obese are more responsive to internal and less responsive to external cues. This evidence supports the notion that there are different types or patterns of obesity and that early-onset obesity may be more related to disturbances in biological set point.

Milich [59] conducted an investigation to compare and contrast Schacter's and Singh's theories. The results failed to confirm either theory; however, the importance of determining the impact of specific variables (e.g., degree of obesity, age of onset, and cue responsiveness) on the behavior of obese individuals was reinforced. Rodin et al. [25] proposed that the predisposition to external stimuli should be measured before attempting to manipulate external cues.

As the external cue theory was evolving, Herman and Mack [60] introduced the concept of restrained eating, linking it to Schacter's theory. The use of the Restrained Eating Questionnaire [61] revealed that low restrained eaters ate in conformity to Schacter's characterization of normal weight individuals (i.e., internal regulation). Further, highly restrained normal weight individuals behaved in an external style; however, once their restraint was gone, they overate. This evidence suggested that some normal weight people overcome the biological set point and reduce their weight through restrained eating. Consequently, it has become apparent that there is no reason to classify all obese people as external and all normal weight people as internal; it is necessary to measure the degree of cue responsiveness and restraint.

Hawkins and Clement [44] pursued this connection even further, relating these issues to binge eating tendencies. More severe binge eating problems were associated with stringent attempts at restrained eating. Collectively, these results suggest that restraint due to extreme dieting concern leads to a chronic state of deprivation, where individuals may become overly responsive once confronted with food cues. The pattern exhibited is a starvation and binging cycle [62]. This eating style is very important to recognize, particularly the restrained or starvation phase of the cycle, because people tend to focus on the binge phase and the guilt it produces. They overlook the starvation phase and do not realize it is a predisposing factor. The professional should always identify binge eating tendencies as a "red flag" to explore other indications of the "starve/stuff" syndrome, and consequent entry into the self-defeating behavior cycle (Figure 2).

Other obese eating styles have been characterized throughout the years. Stunkard [63] classified three eating patterns:

1. Night eating syndrome—characterized by morning anorexia, evening hyperphagia, and insomnia.
2. Eating binge—evident when large amounts of food are consumed in an orgiastic manner at irregular intervals.
3. Eating without satiation—associated with damage to the central nervous system.

Hartz [7] identified that those individuals who manifested the night eating syndrome had a poor prognosis.

Stunkard and his associates [64,65] concluded that there is an enormous plasticity in obese eating styles and that each must be carefully analyzed. For example, most behavioral intervention programs emphasize reducing the pace of eating; however, Stunkard's work has shown that not all obese individuals eat fast and that some normal weight subjects do.

In evaluating the calories consumed, second portions, cleaning the plate, frequency, and time spent eating, Jeffery et al. [66] found that the obese ate more calories at each meal and more frequent snacks. Krassner et al. [67] observed the amount of food left on plates and identified that the obese left less food on their plates. Gates and Huenemann [68] observed the tendency for obese to select more servings of food and more high-calorie and low-nutrition foods in a cafeteria. At fast food sites, obese individuals were noted to eat more highly palatable foods in large quantities [69].

These investigations demonstrated certain tendencies that should be evaluated: meal and snacking patterns, food choices, rate of eating, and sensitivity to environmental stimuli. The unpredictable nature of individuals, however, makes it necessary to analyze each person's style to identify the situations which present problems. The Eating Behavior Inventory [70] is an instrument which could facilitate this process. Self-reporting methods, particularly the food record, was associated with substantial error when used to assess the food consumption of obese individuals [71]. A 24-hour recall in the form of an interview revealed more reliable estimates and was recommended as a preferred method. Regardless of the technique used, a thorough assessment of eating behavior and the variables associated with obese eating styles is required.

Activity Patterns

Considerably more attention has been given to analyzing eating habits than activity patterns in the obese [49]. In fact, most of the research in the area of physical activity and obesity has been done on children. The work of Mayer and his colleagues [72,73] in the 1950s and 1960s implicated inactivity as the predominant difference in the weight-related behaviors of obese and nonobese children. Despite this early evidence, exercise has not been investigated as extensively as eating behavior.

The methods for assessing calorie expenditure from activity include self report, laboratory supervised exercise regimens,

Table 8.   Approximate Energy Cost of Various Exercises
and Sports

Sport or exercise	Total calories expended per minute of activity
Climbing	10.7-13.2
Cycling 5.5 mph	4.5
9.4 mph	7.0
13.1 mph	1.1
Dancing	3.3-7.7
Football	8.9
Golf	5.0
Gymnastics	
Balancing	2.5
Abdominal exercises	3.0
Trunk bending	3.5
Arms swinging, hopping	6.5
Rowing 51 str./min.	4.1
87 str./min.	7.0
97 str./min.	11.2
Running	
Short-distance	13.3-16.6
Cross-country	10.6
Tennis	7.1
Skating (fast)	11.5
Skiing, moderate speed	10.8-15.9
Uphill, maximum speed	18.6
Squash	10.2
Swimming	
Breaststroke	11.0
Backstroke	11.5
Crawl (55 yd./min.)	14.0
Wrestling	14.2

unsupervised prescribed activity programs, pedometers, and observations in the natural environment [49]. Another approach is to look up the caloric cost of various activities, which can be obtained from several sources [74–76] (Table 8). After determining the minutes spent in each activity throughout the day, calculation of the daily energy expenditure is possible with the help of these tables. An individual's overall level of activity could also be approximated by scoring or measuring the following forms of activity:

1. *Lifestyle habits*—tabulating use of stairs, walking for transportation, labor saving devices.
2. *Occupation*—categorizing it as sedentary, active, or strenuous.
3. *Recreational*—determining the frequency and type of sports activities.
4. *Fitness Routine*—evaluating the frequency, time, intensity, and type of fitness activities.

This approach to assessing activity levels may not yield accurate appraisal of calorie expenditure; however, it can be useful for comparing baseline and post-treatment activity patterns. If the intervention process promotes lifestyle changes in exercise habits, it would be important to consider these factors in evaluating the impact of treatment.

For example, Brownell et al. [77] conducted an interesting observation study to determine the effect of posting a sign at the bottom of a staircase in a shopping mall to encourage the use of stairs, instead of escalators. Posting the sign significantly increased the use of stairs, indicating that increased awareness may account for behavior change.

The techniques mentioned here are all estimates of activity level, and thus of calorie expenditure. None of these approaches account for individual variations in metabolic rate. Determination of total energy expenditure can be accomplished only by using direct or indirect calorimetry, both of which are very costly, complicated, and impractical procedures [49].

In summary, appraisal of activity patterns is a critical component of comprehensive assessment. It is no less important than eating behavior analysis even though it has not been emphasized as much. Consideration should be given to all aspects of a person's life in assessing the level of activity.

CONCLUSIONS

Comprehensive assessment of the interrelated variables determining the state of obesity has been recognized as a critical precursor to treatment. Brownell [49] presented a comprehensive

Table 9.

Target	Methods	Advantages	Disadvantages	Preferred method(s)
		Physiology		
Adipose cellularity (size)	Microscopic assessment	Economy, simplicity	Measurement error	Microscopic measurement or electronic count
	Optical measurement of collagenase-treated tissue	Economy, simplicity	Measurement error	
	Electronic count of osmium-fixed cells	Many cells are counted, small error	Cost, toxicity risk, exclusion of small cells	
Adipose cellularity	Calculation from average cell size and total body fat (no direct methods available)	Simplicity	Multiplication of measurement error	Calculation from average cell size determined from four areas
Physical status Endocrine Hypothalamic Cardiopulmonary Orthopedic Genetic Weight history Family history	Standard physiologic assessment	Specific to method	Specific to method	Algorithm by Bray et al. (1976)
Body fat	Carcass composition	Less error, direct measurement	Cost, difficulty	Body-mass index plus skinfold thickness
	Height-weight subtraction	Simplicity, economy	Calculation error, measurement error ?Relation to body fat	
	Broca index	Simplicity, economy		
	Magic 36	Simplicity, economy		
	Ruler test	Simplicity, economy		
	Eyeball test	Simplicity, economy		
	Height-weight tables	Simplicity, economy	Large error	

Body weight	Weight/height	Simplicity, economy	?Relation to body fat	
	Body-mass index	Simplicity, economy	?Relation to body fat	
	Skinfold thickness	Economy, validity	Poor reliability	
	Body circumference	Economy, validity	Sophisticated analyses	
	Somatyping	Economy	?Relation to body fat	
	Hydrostatic weighing	Accuracy	Cost	
	Weighing on scale	Accuracy	None	
	Self-report	Accuracy	Subject to distortion	Weighing, self-report
	Naturalistic observation	Nonobtrusive, economy	?Reliability, validity	
Eating behaviors				
	Food choice	Measurable in natural settings	? of inference to hunger	
Environment responsivity	Ad libitum food after manipulation of cue salience	Can alter cue salience and study in laboratory	Inference from independent variable, reactivity, artificial situation	Mahoney Master Questionnaire
	Mahoney Master Questionnaire	Economy, psychometric evaluation	Validity untested, potential distortion	
	Eating Patterns Questionnaire	Economy	Never validated	
Restrained eating	Herman Scale	Economy, brevity, general use	Validity untested, potential distortion	Herman Questionnaire
	Stunkard Scale	Economy, psychometric evaluation	Further evaluation of validity needed, potential distortion	Stunkard Questionnaire

(Continued)

Table 9. (Continued)

Physical activity

Target	Methods	Advantages	Disadvantages	Preferred method(s)
Total energy expenditure (direct measurement)	Direct calorimetry (heat loss from controlled chamber)	Direct and total measure, no error, control of environment	Cost, not practical for humans	Direct calorimetry
Total energy expenditure (indirect measurement)	Metabolic rate calculated from oxidation values	Somewhat precise	Error in measurement, cost, obtrusiveness	Heart rate
	Water vaporization from lungs	Good correlation with total energy expenditure	Error in measurement, cost, obtrusiveness	
	Heart rate	Accuracy	Cost, obtrusiveness, subject to extraneous influence	
Programmed exercise	Self-report	Economy, continuous measure, simplicity	?Validity and reactivity, possible distortion and error in measurement	Pedometer for measure of magnitude, direct observation and heart-rate recording for intensity
	Direct observation	Validity and low measurement error	?Reactivity, cost, obtrusiveness	
	Motion picture sampling	Reliability, possibly high validity	?Reactivity, cost, obtrusiveness	
	Pedometer	Economy, simplicity, fairly high accuracy	Mechanical malfunction, ?reactivity, cannot measure intensity	
	Heart-rate recording	Accuracy	Cost, obtrusiveness, subject to extraneous influences	

	Method	Advantages	Disadvantages	Instruments
Routine exercise	Self-report	Economy, continuous measure, simplicity	?Validity and reactivity, possible distortion and error in measurement	Pedometer
	Naturalistic observation	Economy, nonobtrusive	Difficult to track individuals, ?generalizability	
	Pedometer	Economy, simplicity, fairly high accuracy	Mechanical malfunction, ?reactivity	
	Heart-rate recording	Accuracy	Cost, obtrusiveness, subject to extraneous influences	

Psychological and social adjustment

	Method	Advantages	Disadvantages	Instruments
Psychological functioning	Self-report	Economy, allows questioning	Potential distortion	Beck Depression Inventory, Mahoney Master Questionnaire, SCL-90, self-report, report from others
	Reports from family or friend	Allows view of "real world" behavior, economy	Accuracy and potential distortion	
	Beck Depression Inventory Symptom Checklist (SCL-90)	Economy, validated, easy to administer frequently	Measures only depression, potential distortion	
		Economy, measures several areas of functioning, validated	Potential distortion	
	MMPI	Validated psychometric evaluation, general use	Potential distortion, somewhat difficult to score	
	Mahoney Master Questionnaire	Measures psychological responses specific to obesity, measures cognitive behavior, psychometric evaluation	Validity untested, potential distortion	

(Continued)

Table 9. (Continued)

Target	Methods	Advantages	Disadvantages	Preferred method(s)
Social functioning	Self-report	Economy, allows questioning	Potential distortion	Marital Adjustment Test, self-report, report from others
	Reports from family or friend	Allows view of "real world" behavior, economy	Accuracy and potential distortion	
	Locke-Wallace Marital Adjustment Test	Validated, economy, simplicity, interpretability, can be completed by partner	Potential distortion, measures only one facet of adjustment	
	Other adjustment inventories	Economy, simplicity	Potential distortion, ?validity	
Independent variables (adherence)				
Dietary change	Self-report	Economy, simplicity	?Reactivity, potential distortion, error in measurement	Self-report with collaboration from others
	Reports from family or friend	Substantiates self-report, economy	Error in measurement, potential distortion	
	Nutrition survey	Economy, simplicity	Potential distortion, error in measurement	
	Blood or urine analysis	Accuracy	Cost, obtrusiveness, subject to extraneous influences	

Dimension	Measure	Advantages	Disadvantages	Recommended
Prescribed behaviors	Self-report	Economy, simplicity	?Reactivity, potential distortion, error in measurement	Self-report with collaboration from others
	Reports from family or friend	Substantiates self-report, economy	Error in measurement, potential distortion	
	Mahony Master Questionnaire	Economy, psychometric evaluation	Validity untested, potential distortion	
Treatment outcome				
Weight change	Absolute weight change	Simplicity, economy, accuracy, general use	Ignores body fat, body size	Weight-reduction quotient, absolute weight change
	Change in percentage overweight	Simplicity, economy, accuracy, accounts for ideal weight	?Norms, ignores body fat	
	Categorical weight loss	Economy, general use, accuracy	Ignores body fat, body size, sex, and variability	
	Weight-reduction quotient	Economy, accuracy, accounts for ideal body weight and surplus weight, increasing general use	Ignores body fat	
Medical change				
Blood pressure	Pressure cuff	Economy, general use	Some measurement error	Medical practices in use
Plasma lipids	Lipid analysis	Accuracy	Cost, obtrusiveness	
Glucose tolerance	Tolerance test	Accuracy	Cost, obtrusiveness	
Cardiac efficiency	Stress test	Accuracy	Cost, obtrusiveness	

From Brownell, K. D. Assessment of Eating Disorders, in *Behavioral Assessment of Adult Disorders.* Guilford Press, New York, 1981, p. 366–376.

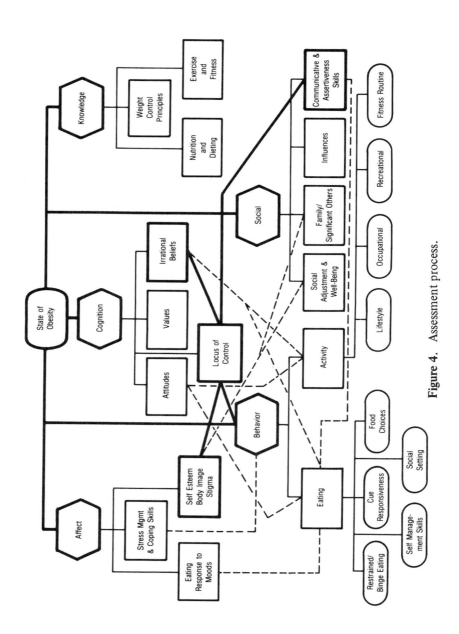

Figure 4. Assessment process.

assessment plan (Table 9) which outlines both physiological and behavioral factors. This plan describes the advantages and disadvantages of available techniques for assessing these factors.

The issues discussed in this chapter are broad in scope, yet have very apparent connections. An ideal assessment process would consolidate and cross-reference these variables to elicit patterns in cognitions, affect, and behavior. Figure 4 diagrammatically illustrates a conceptual model for comprehensive, behavior analysis of eating and activity patterns. A standardized evaluation system of this nature would enhance our understanding of obesity, facilitate research efforts, and improve the intervention process.

REFERENCES

1. Granat, J. P. Obesity: a family problem. *Obesity/Bariatric Medicine* 8:178-180, 1979.
2. Greenberg, I., Palambo, J. D., and Blackburn, G. L. Obesity: Facts, fads, and fantasies. *Comprehensive Therapy* 5:68-76, 1979.
3. Marston, A. R., London, P., Cooper, L. M., and Lammas, S. E. Lifestyle: a behavioral program for weight reduction and obesity research. *Obesity/Bariatric Medicine* 5:95-100, 1976.
4. Reich, L. A., and Pion, L. A. The management of obesity through self centered behavior change. *Journal of Reproductive Medicine* 22:1-43, 1979.
5. Brownell, K. Obesity: Understanding and treating a serious, prevalent, and refractory disorder. *Journal of Consulting and Clinical Psychology* 50:820-840, 1982.
6. Blackburn, G. Multidisciplinary approach to adult obesity therapy. *International Journal of Obesity* 2:133-142, 1978.
7. Hartz, A. J., Kalkhoff, R. K., Rimm, A. A., and McCall, R. J. A study of factors associated with the ability to maintain weight loss. *Preventative Medicine* 8:471-483, 1979.
8. Leon, G. L. Personality and morbid obesity—Implications for dietary management through behavior modification. *Surgical Clinics of North America* 59:1007-1015, 1979.
9. Setty, R. M., and Hawkins, R. C. Factors predicting success in a broad spectrum behavioral weight control program after treatment and at follow-up. American Psychological Association Annual Convention, 1980.

10. Wise, T. N., and Fernandez, F. Psychological profiles of candidates seeking surgical correction for obesity. *Obesity/Bariatric Medicine 8*: 83-86, 1979.

11. Kotkov, B., and Murawski, B. A Rorschach study of the personality structure of obese women. *Journal of Clinical Psychology 8*:391-396, 1952.

12. Hewitt, M. I., O'Dell, D. S., Schellas, K. P., and Kotnour, K. D. Predictability of patient compliance with a weight reduction program. *Obesity/Bariatric Medicine 6*:218-221, 1977.

13. Young, C. M., Berresford, K., and Moore, N. S. Psychological factors in weight control. *American Journal of Clinical Nutrition 5*:186-191, 1957.

14. Perelberg, H., Neil, S. E., Kahans, D., Soccio, M. G., and Costa, R. A. Personality of a group of grossly obese women. *Australian and New Zealand Journal of Psychiatry 12*:297-299, 1978.

15. Grinker, J. Behavioral and metabolic consequences of weight reduction. *Journal of the American Dietetic Association 62*:30-34., 1973.

16. Schumaker, J. F., Wagner, M. K., Grodnitzky, B. H., and Lockwood, G. E. Eating behaviors and psychotherapy approaches to weight reduction. *Obesity/Bariatric Medicine 5*:136-139, 1976.

17. Jordon, H. A., Kimbrell, G. M., and Levitz, L. S. Managing obesity—Why diet is not enough. *Postgraduate Medicine 59*:183-186, 1976.

18. Straw, M., Mahoney, M. J., Straw, R. B., Rogers, T., and Stunkard, A. J. A self-report measure of variables relevant to obesity treatment. *Addictive Behaviors*, 1984, in press.

19. Rotter, J. B. Some problems and misconceptions related to the construct of internal versus external control of reinforcement. *Journal of Consulting and Clinical Psychology 43*:56-57, 1975.

20. O'Bryan, G. The relationship between an individual's I-E orientation and information-seeking, learning, and use of weight control relevant information. *Dissertation Abstracts International 33*B:447B (University Microfilms No. 72-19:541), 1972.

21. Rotter, J. B. Generalized expectancies for internal versus external control of reinforcement. *Psychological Monographs 80*:(whole No. 609), 1966.

22. Craddock, K. D. Psychological and personality factors associated with successful weight reduction: a 10-year follow-up of 134 personal cases. In: A. Howard (ed.), *Recent Advances in Obesity Research.* Newman Publishing, London, 1975.

23. Leon, G. R. Personality, body image, and eating pattern changes in overweight persons after weight loss. In: A Howard (ed.), *Recent Advances in Obesity Research.* Newman Publishing, London, 1975.

24. Ley, P., Bradshaw, P. W., Kincey, J. A., Couper-Smartt, J., and Wilson, M. Psychological variables in the control of obesity. In: W. L. Burland, P. Samuel, and J. Yudkin (eds.), *Obesity Symposium—Servier Research Institute*. Churchhill and Livingstone, London, 1975.

25. Rodin, J., Bray, G. A., Atkinson, R. L., Dahms, W. T., Greenway, F. L., Hamilton, K., and Molitch, M. Predictors of successful weight loss in an outpatient obesity clinic. *International Journal of Obesity* 1:79-87.

26. Tobias, L. L., and McDonald, M. L. Internal locus of control and weight loss: an insufficient condition. *Journal of Consulting and Clinical Psychology 45*:647-653, 1977.

27. Ellis, A. *Reason and Emotion in Psychotherapy*. Lyle Stuart, New York, 1962.

28. Ellis, A., and Harper, R. A. *A New Guide to Rational Living*. Wilshire Book Co., North Hollywood, CA, 1979.

29. Morelli, G. Cognitive Rumination: A barrier to behavioral compliance. *Obesity/Bariatric Medicine 8*:118-119, 1979.

30. Leon, G. R. Cognitive-Behavior Therapy for Eating Disturbances. In: P. Kendall and S. Hollon (eds.), *Cognitive-Behavioral Interventions: Theory, Research and Procedures*. Academic Press, Inc., New York, 1979.

31. Foreyt, J., and Goodrick, G. K. Weight disorders. In: C. J. Golden, S. Strider, and B. Graber (eds.), *Applied Techniques in Behavioral Medicine*. Grune and Stratton, New York, 1971.

32. Osman, J. D. *Thin from Within*. New York, Hart Publishing Company, 1976.

33. Summerskill, J., and Darling, C. D. Emotional adjustment and dieting performance, *Journal of Consulting Psychology 19*:151-153, 1955.

34. Gold, D. Psychological factors associated with obesity. *American Family Physician 13*:87-91, 1976.

35. Leon, G. R., and Chamberlain, K. Comparison of daily eating habits and emotional states of overweight persons successful or unsuccessful in maintaining weight loss. *Journal of Consulting and Clinical Psychology 41*:108-115, 1973.

36. Hewitt, M. I. Negative mood, hunger and weight classification. *Obesity/Bariatric Medicine 3*:24-27, 1974.

37. Kalisch, B. The stigma of obesity. *American Journal of Nursing 72*:1124-1127, 1972.

38. Allon, N. Self-perceptions of the stigma of overweight in relationship to weight-losing patterns. *American Journal of Clinical Nutrition 32*:470-480, 1979.

39. Craft, C. A. Body image and obesity. *Nursing Clinics of North America 7*:77-85, 1972.

40. Stunkard, A. J., and Rush, J. Dieting and depression reexamined: A critical view of reports of ontoward responses during weight reduction for obesity. *Annals of Internal Medicine 81*:526-533, 1974.

41. Tobias, A. L., and Gordon, J. B. Social consequences of obesity. *Journal of the American Dietetic Association 76*:388-342, 1980.

42. Krantz, D. S. A naturalistic study of social influences on meal size among moderately obese and nonobese subjects. *Psychosomatic Medicine 41*:19-27, 1979.

43. Rosenthal, B. S., and Marx, R. D. Determinants of initial relapse episodes among dieters. *Obesity/Bariatric Medicine 10*:94-97, 1981.

44. Hawkins, R. C., and Clement, P. F. Development and validation of a self-report measure of binge eating tendencies. *Addictive Behaviors 5*: 219-226, 1980.

45. Galassi, J. P., DeLo, J. S., Galassi, M. D., and Bastien, S. The college self-expression scale: a measure of assertiveness. *Behavior Therapy 5*: 165-171, 1974.

46. Granat, J. P. Obesity: a family problem. *Obesity/Bariatric Medicine 8*:178-180, 1979.

49. Brownell, K. D. Assessment of Eating Disorders. In: D. Barlow, *Behavioral Assessment of Adult Disorders.* Guilford Press, New York, 1981.

50. Schacter, S. Obesity and eating. *Science 161*:751-761, 1968.

51. Schacter, S., Goldman, R., and Gordon, A. Effects of fear, food deprivation, and obesity on eating. *Journal of Personality and Social Psychology 10*:91-97, 1968.

52. Stunkard, A. J. Environment and obesity: Recent advances in our understanding of regulation of food intake in man. *Federation Proceedings 27*:1368-1373, 1968.

53. Nisbett, R. E. Taste, deprivation, and weight determinants of eating behavior. *Journal of Personality and Social Psychology 10*:107-116, 1968.

47. Kohrs, M. B. The association of obesity with socioeconomic factors in Missouri. *American Journal of Clinical Nutrition 32*:2120-2128, 1979.

48. Zegman, M., and Baker, B. Relationship between weight loss and changes in eating habits, exercise, and caloric intake during and after a behavioral weight control program. Paper presented at the Association for Advancement of Behavior Therapy, Los Angeles, CA, 1982.

54. Schacter, S., and Gross, L. Eating and the manipulation of time. *Journal of Personality and Social Psychology 10*:98–106, 1968.

55. Nisbett, R. E. Determinants of food intake in obesity. *Science 159*: 1254–1255, 1968.

56. Schacter, S. Some extraordinary facts about obese humans and rats. *American Psychologist 26*:129–144, 1971.

57. Singh, D., Swanson, J., Letz, R., and Sanders, M. Performance of obese humans on transfer of training and reaction time tasks. *Psychosomatic Medicine 35*:240–249, 1973.

58. Wagner, M. K., and Schumaker, J. F. External-cue responsivity in obese children. *Obesity/Bariatric Medicine 5*:168–169, 1976.

59. Milich, R. S., and Fisher, E. B. Effects of cue salience and prior training on the behavior of juvenile- and adult-onset obese individuals. *Addictive Behaviors 4*:1–10, 1979.

60. Herman, C. P., and Mack, D. Restrained and unrestrained eating. *Journal of Personality 43*:647–660, 1975.

61. Herman, C. P., and Polivy, J. Anxiety, restraint and eating behavior. *Journal of Abnormal Psychology 84*:666–672, 1975.

62. Leon, G. R., Roth, L., and Hewitt, M. I. Eating patterns, satiety, and self-control behavior of obese persons during weight reduction. *Obesity/Bariatric Medicine 6*:172–181, 1977.

63. Stunkard, A. J. Eating patterns and obesity. *Psychiatric Quarterly 33*: 284–295, 1959.

64. Stunkard, A. J., and Kaplan, D. Eating in public places: a review of reports of the direct observation of eating behavior. *International Journal of Obesity 1*:89–101, 1977.

65. Adams, N., Ferguson, J., Stunkard, A. J., and Agras, S. Eating behaviors of obese and nonobese women. *Behavior Research and Therapy 16*:225–232, 1978.

66. Wing, R. R., Carrol, C., and Jeffrey, R. W. Repeated observation of obese and normal subjects eating in the natural environment. *Addictive Behaviors 3*:191–196, 1978.

67. Krassner, H. A., Brownell, K. D., and Stunkard, A. J. Cleaning the plate: food left by overweight and normal weight persons. *Behavior Research and Therapy 17*:155–156, 1979.

68. Gates, J. C., Huenemann, R. L., and Brand, R. J. Food choices of obese and non-obese persons. *Journal of the American Dietetic Association 67*:339–343, 1975.

69. Coll, M., Meyer, A., and Stunkard, A. J. Obesity and food choices in public places. *Archives of General Psychiatry 36*:795–797, 1979.

70. O'Neil, P. M., Currey, H. S., Hirsch, A. A., Malcolm, R. J., Sexauer, J. D., Riddle, F. E., and Taylor, C. I. Development and validation of the Eating Behavior Inventory. *Journal of Behavior Assessment 1*: 123-132, 1979.

71. Lansky, D., and Brownell, K. D. Estimates of food quantities: errors in self-report among obese patients. *American Journal of Clinical Nutrition 35*:727-732, 1982.

72. Johnson, M. T., Burke, B. S., and Mayer, J. Relative importance of inactivity and overeating in the energy balance of obese high school girls. *American Journal of Clinical Nutrition 4*:33-44, 1956.

73. Bullen, B. A., Reed, R. B., and Mayer, J. Physical activity of obese and non-obese adolescent girls appraised by motion picture sampling. *American Journal of Clinical Nutrition 14*:211-223, 1964.

74. Stuart, R. B., and Davis, B. *Slim Chance in a Fat World: Behavioral Control of Obesity*. Research Press, Champaign, IL, 1972.

75. Getchell, B. *Being Fit: A Personal Guide*. John Wiley and Sons, Inc., New York, 1982.

76. American Alliance of Health, Physical Education, and Recreation. *Nutrition for Athletes—A Handbook for Coaches*. Washington, D.C., 1971.

77. Brownell, K. D., Stunkard, A. J., and Albaum, J. M. Evaluation and modification of exercise patterns in the natural environment. *American Journal of Psychiatry 137*:1540-1545, 1980.

Index

Abdominal skinfold measurements,
    99, 100, 102, 103, 106–107
Addictive behavior, 85
Adipocytes, 27–29
Adipose tissue, 23, 27
Aerobic activity, 32–33
Affect, 128–132
Aging and body density, 97, 99
Alpha-amylase inhibitors, 11
Amitriptyline, 87
Amphetamines, 10
Anger, 128, 131
Anthropometric measurements
    of body composition, 93–94
    in body density prediction,
        94–96
    in clinical assessment of obesity,
        72–73
    descriptive statistics for, 100
Antidepressants, 86, 87
Antigens, HLA, 78
Antipsychotics, 86, 87
Anxiety
    oral activity and, 128
    weight control and, 86

Appetite
    exercise affecting, 33
    medications suppressing, 10–11
Assertiveness skills, 132
Assessment of obesity, 71–92
    anthropometric and body
        measurements, 72–73
    associated diseases, 73
    developmental history, 78–81
    diet and meal pattern, 81–82
    family history, 77–78
    medications, 86–87
    metabolic rate, 73–77
    personality, 85
    physical activity pattern, 82–83
    psychiatric disturbances, 86
    response to external cues, 83
    restrained eating, 83–84

Basal metabolic rate, 73–74
Behavior
    activity pattern and, 137–139
    eating. See Eating behavior
    irrational beliefs and, 122–126
    locus of control in, 120–122

[Behavior]
motivation in control of,
130
self-defeating, 121, 122
values affecting, 126–128
weight-related, 134–139
Behavior therapy
for adult-onset obesity, 114
cognitive approaches to, 16–21
Bell Adjustment Inventory, 114
Benzodiazepines, 86–87
Binge eating behavior, 136
Blood pressure, high. *See* Hypertension
Body circumferences
in body density prediction
equations, 93, 94–96
in population specific equations
of body fat, 96–97
Body composition measurements,
93–110
generalized equations for, 97–
109
height–weight, 94–96
interpretation of, 110
population specific equations
for, 96–97
Body density, 93, 94
accuracy of measurements of,
102
aging and, 97, 99
generalized equations for, 94,
97–109
population specific equations
for, 94, 96–97
skinfold thickness measurements
and, 97–99
Body diameters, 93, 96
Body fat, 23
anthropometric variables for
prediction of, 94–96
of athletes, 110
in developmental history, 79–
80

[Body fat]
estimation of percentage of, 72,
94
for men, 106–107
for women, 108–109
familial trends in, 78
optimal levels of, 110
weight of, 94
Body image, 114
Body measurements, 72–73
Body weight. *See* Weight
Bone weight, 94

Calorie expenditure for physical
activity, 137–139
Calorie management, 4
basal metabolic rate and, 73–74,
77
via diet. *See* Diet
education on, 119
Carbohydrates
amitriptyline causing cravings
for, 87
in diabetes, 51
in hypertension, 59, 60
triiodothyronine and, 76, 77
Cardiovascular disease, 1, 2, 47–48
Cattel Neuroticism Scale, 114
Central nervous system, 6, 47
Chest skinfold measurements, 99,
100, 102, 103, 106–107
Chlordiazepoxide, 86–87
Cholesterol
in fat, 27
in hypercholesterolemia, 54–56
Chorionic gonadotropin, human, 11
Cognitive processes in obesity, 120–
128
behavior therapy based on, 16–21
factors affecting, 120
irrational beliefs, 122–126
locus of control, 120–122
values, 126–128
Communication skills, 128, 132

Coping skills, 132
Coronary artery disease, 1, 47
Cost factors in weight control pro-
grams, 133–134
Cultural factors
in bias against obesity, 2, 17
in eating behavior, 7, 35–36
Cushing's disease, 73

Defensiveness, 128
Depression, 86
Diabetes
cholesterol levels in, 56
insulin resistance in, 49–50
insulin secretion in, 48–49
obesity and, 1, 47, 73
treatment of, 50–54
with diet, 51–52
with exercise, 52–53
with insulin, 50–51
Diazepam, 86–87
Diets
assessment of patient knowledge
of, 119
depression from, 86
in diabetes treatment, 51–52
evaluation of, 81–82
affecting fat deposition, 33–35
in hypercholesterolemia treatment, 56
in hypertension treatment, 60–61
metabolic rate and, 75–77
misinformation on, 118
for obesity treatment, 14–15
success rates for, 15
Drugs
food consumption changes from,
86–87
weight loss, 10–11

Eating Behavior Inventory, 137
Eating behavior
binge, 136
biological factors in, 5–6

[Eating behavior]
cue responsiveness in, 134–135
environmental factors in, 6
evaluation of, 81–82
negative moods and, 131
restrained, 83–84
therapy choice based on, 114
Education
level of, vs predisposition to
obesity, 132
nutrition, 114
of weight control principles,
13–14, 116–119
Elavil, 87
Emotional disturbances of obesity,
128–131
Energy balance
cause of, 71–72
regulation of, 5–9, 23–38
biological determinants in, 5–7
immediate environment
determinants, 9
macrosocial and experiential
determinants, 7–9
Energy costs of exercise, 138
Environment
cognitive processes affected by,
120
cues in, for eating, 83, 134–135
in energy balance, 9
weight influenced by, 25, 35–37
Evolution and eating behavior, 6
Exercise
assessment of knowledge of principles of, 118
in diabetes treatment, 52–53
energy cost of, 138
in hypertension management, 60
misconceptions of, 123
weight loss from, 32–33

Family
eating behaviors influenced by,
7–8

[Family]
negative influence of, on weight loss, 132
weight trends within, 24, 77–78
Fat
body. *See* Body fat
dietary factors affecting deposition of, 33–35
Fat cells, 27–29
Food
choices and preferences for, 134, 137
diets. *See* Diets
emotional needs satisfied by, 8
social adjustment and, 128
stigma attached to specific types of, 20

Gastric surgery, 12, 54, 56
Gastrointestinal factors in eating behavior, 6
Genetic factors in weight, 24–25
Glucagon, 52
Growth hormone, 26
Guilt, 131, 133

Height–weight measurements, 45, 46, 94–96
Hereditary factors in obesity, 24–25
Hormones
eating behavior and, 6
glucagon, 52
growth, 26
human chorionic gonadotropin, 11
insulin, 26, 48–51, 58–60
in obesity treatment, 11
thyroid, 76, 77
Hostility, 128
Human chorionic gonadotropin, 11
Hypercholesterolemia, 54–56
Hyperlipidemia, 73
Hyperphagia, 25

Hypertension
obesity and, 1, 47, 73
sodium intake and, 56–57, 60
weight loss for management of, 56–61
Hypoglycemic agents, oral, 53
Hypothalamus, 25–27

Ileojejunal bypass operation, 11
Income vs obesity, 133
Insulin, 26
in hypertension, 58–60
in pathogenesis of diabetes, 48–50
in treatment of diabetes, 50–51
Irrational beliefs, 123
Isotopic dilution, 93

Jaw wiring, 12

Ketosis, 119
Knowledge Test, 117

Laurence–Moon–Bardet–Biedl syndrome, 73
Laxatives in weight control, 12–13
Leikert Scale, 127
Librium, 86–87
Lifestyle
activity pattern and, 137–139
eating behavior and, 8–9, 134–137
Lithium, 87
Locus of control construct, 120–122
Love and affection, 130

Malabsorption syndrome, 11
Master Questionnaire, 117
Media in weight control, 13, 134
Medications
food consumption changes due to, 86–87
for weight loss, 10–11

Metabolism
    basal rate of, 73–74
    exercise affecting, 32–33
MMPI, 114
Mortality ratios, 43–47
Motivation, 129–130
Muscle weight, 94

Night eating syndrome, 136
Norepinephrine, 57–60
Nowlis Mood Checklist, 114
Nutrition
    assessment of, 81–82, 119
    eating behavior and, 6
    education on, 114
    faddism, 123

Obesity
    in cause of death, 47–48
    central vs peripheral, 73
    clinical assessment of. *See*
        Assessment of obesity
    as crime, 18
    cultural bias against, 2, 17
    discrimination against, 17–18
    as disease, 18
    emotional disturbances and,
        128–134
    as health risk factor, 1
    hypertrophic vs hyperplastic, 28,
        78–80
    incidence of, 1
    level of education and income
        vs, 133
    mortality rates with, 43–47
    psychological factors associated
        with, 16–18, 113–147
    stigma attached to, 17–21
    thermogenic response to food
        intake in, 77
    urban vs rural areas and, 133
    weight loss for. *See* Weight loss
Obesity tissue, 23
Overweight, 23
Oxygen consumption, 74

Personality Factor Questionnaire,
    114
Personality, 85
Phenylpropanolamine, 10
Phospholipids, 27
Physical activity
    in appetite suppression, 33
    assessment of patterns of, 82–83,
        137–139, 142–143
    in weight control, 13, 14, 32–33
Physical fitness concepts, 118
Potassium-40, 93
Prader–Willi syndrome, 73
Psychiatric disturbances, 86
Psychological factors in obesity,
    16–17, 113–147
    affect, 128–132
    assessment of, 113–116, 143–
        144
    cognitive processes, 120–128
        irrational beliefs, 122–126
        locus of control, 120–122
        values, 126–128
    knowledge of weight control
        principles and, 116–119
    social influences, 132–134
    weight-related behaviors, 134–
        139
        activity patterns, 137–139
        eating habits, 134–137
Psychotherapy, 114
Purging, 12–13

Radiographic analysis, 93
Rational-emotive therapy, 122–
    126
Religious views of obesity, 17–18
Repression, 128
Restrained Eating Questionnaire,
    138
Rorschach test, 114

SCL-90, 114
Self-defeating behavior cycle, 121,
    122

Self-esteem
    inadequacy and, 131
    obesity affecting, 17
Self-rejection, 126
Set point concept of weight regula-
    tion, 29-32
Skinfold thickness measurements,
    72, 93
    abdomen, 99, 100, 102, 103,
      106-107
    in body density prediction equa-
      tions, 94-96
      generalized, 97-109
      population specific, 96-97
    chest, 99, 100, 102, 103, 106-
      107
    suprailium, 99, 100, 102, 105,
      108-109
    thigh, 99, 100, 102, 104, 106-
      109
    triceps, 99, 100, 102, 104, 108-
      109
Social factors affecting weight, 35-
    37, 132-134, 143-144
Sociocultural interventions for
    obesity treatment, 13-14
Socioeconomic factors in obesity,
    133
Sodium retention, 56-60
Somatotyping, 73
Sports, 139
Starch blockers, 11
Sucrose, 34-35
Suprailium skinfold measurements,
    99, 100, 102, 105, 108-
    109
Surgery in obesity treatment, 11

Taste, 6
Thigh skinfold measurements, 99,
    100, 102, 103, 106-109
Thyroid disorders, 73
Thyroid hormones, 76, 77
Tranquilizers, 86, 87

Triceps skinfold measurements, 99,
    100, 102, 104, 108-109
Triglycerides, 27
Triiodothyronine, 58, 76

Ultrasound techniques, 93
Underwater weighing, 93

Vagus nerve, 25
Valium, 86-87
Values, 126-128
Volume displacement, 93
Vomiting in weight control, 12-13

Weight
    average, for men, 45
    average, for women, 46
    environmental influence on, 25,
      83, 134-135
    familial trends in, 24, 78
    fat cells and, 27-29
    genetics and, 24-25
    height correlated to, 45, 46, 94-
      96
    hypothalamus affecting, 25-27
    maintenance of, motivation for,
      130
    mechanisms of regulation,
      25-27
    metabolic rate vs, 74-75
    mortality vs, 43-47
    physiologic factors affecting,
      24-33, 140-141
    set point concept in regulation
      of, 29-32
    social/environmental factors
      affecting, 35-37
    socioeconomic factors relating
      to, 133
    tissue components of, 94
Weight loss
    assertiveness skills for, 132
    assessment of knowledge of prin-
      ciples of, 116-119

[Weight loss]
  behavioral cognitive approaches
    to, 16–21
  cost factor in, 133–134
  in diabetes management, 48–54
  diets for, 14–15
  education for, 13–14
  energy balance regulation for,
    5–9
    biological determinants in,
      5-7
    immediate environmental
      determinants in, 9
    macrosocial and experiential
      determinants in, 7–9
  evaluation of, 145
  fat cell size in, 80–81
  goals of, 3
  in hypercholesterolemia treat-
    ment, 54–56

[Weight loss]
  in hypertension treatment, 56–
    61
  interventions for, 10–15
  jaw wiring for, 12
  locus of control for, 120–122
  media in, 13
  medical indications for, 2, 43–69
  medications for, 10–11
  physical activity for, 13, 32–33
  purging for, 12–13
  rational-emotive therapy for, 123
  self-concept and, 131
  surgery for, 11–12
  treatment for, 1–21
  triiodothyronine in, 76
  values in, 126
Willpower, 129

Zucker fatty rat, 30, 32